Pep Up Naturally

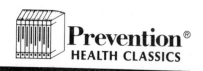

Prevention® **HEALTH CLASSICS**

Pep Up Naturally

by the Editors of Prevention® Magazine

Written and compiled by

Sharon Faelten

With contributions by

Dominick Bosco
Mark Bricklin
Virginia Castleton
Ken Dychtwald, Ph.D.
Jasmine Hope Geyer
William Gottlieb
Charles T. Kuntzleman, Ed.D.
Eileen Mazer

Kerry Pechter
Robert Rodale
Linda Shaw
Porter Shimer
Jonathan Uhlaner
Tom Voss
John Yates

Christy Kohler, Research Associate

Rodale Press, Emmaus, Pennsylvania

NOTICE

The information in this book is designed to help basically healthy people maximize their personal feelings of well-being. The reader should be aware that certain physical ailments, as well as many drugs, can cause fatigue. So can long-lasting emotional problems and overweight. As such, if you suspect that you are experiencing more than a simple lack of pep, we suggest that you seek medical advice.

Books series design by Barbara Field.
Illustrations by Susan Rosenberger.

Library of Congress Cataloging in Publication Data

Main entry under title:
Pep up naturally.
    (Prevention health classics)
    Includes index.
    1. Health. 2. Vitality. I. Faelten, Sharon.
II. Prevention (Emmaus, Pa.) III. Series.
RA776.5.P44   613   81-17783
ISBN 0-87857-379-8 paperback   AACR2

2 4 6 8 10 9 7 5 3 1 paperback

Contents

Introduction

We all have days when we'd like to feel fresher and more energetic. Sometimes an exceptionally long workday or a sleepless night can leave you temporarily pooped. Nothing a little sleep won't cure, though. What's really irksome is a persistent lack of pep, a general listlessness that keeps you feeling only half alive day after day. Sure, you get things done, but it seems to take all the effort you can muster. Maybe you're a tornado of activity all day, only to slip into a fast fade when you hit home. Or perhaps you find yourself putting things off or hesitating to start new projects.

Such fatigue may be accompanied by endless insomnia, a hefty case of "nerves," or inability to concentrate. Yet a medical checkup rules out a sluggish thyroid, high blood pressure, an infection and any other condition that could possibly account for your fatigue. But even when the doctor says there's "nothing wrong" with you, you *know* you could be getting more output from your body and mind.

Well, there are no quick and easy answers, no magic potions to cure that kind of hard-to-pin-down but very real fatigue. But there *is* a personal formula—a program for more energy—that you can evolve for yourself from the suggestions discussed in this book. You may not be aware, for instance, that coffee and other widely used stimulants can actually wear you out instead of pep you up. So we'll show you other ways to perk up—habits that will help you wake up feeling fresher—and stay fresh long into the evening. We'll also talk about some of the other new habits that program may include, such as eating the right foods at the right times to keep your blood sugar levels from seesawing up and down, and enjoying short relaxation breaks to dissolve tension. Plus, you'll find out why it helps to get enough iron and other nutrients that are essential to peak energy, and that regular exercise is a *must* if you want to feel invigorated.

Best of all, perhaps, you'll learn how to overcome boredom and make time for fun in your life, two critical components in a truly active, high-energy life.

Don't feel compelled to try everything in the book at once. Keep in mind that it may have taken years to develop some of the personal habits that are sapping your energy. Try to investigate and develop no more than two or three changes a week. You may be surprised at how soon you feel a real difference in energy levels—a lifetime increase that comes not from without but from a reawakening of your own inner vitality.

PART I

Take Action against Fatigue

Wake Up Feeling Fresher

CHAPTER 1

Each new morning, it's said, is the first day of the rest of your life.

But if that's true, it certainly doesn't help matters any to wake up feeling like you're glued to the bed, or with the suspicion that you've just snapped out of a week-long coma. Or, perhaps most commonly, you feel utter disbelief that it's morning already.

You may also have an aching back. Or a stiff neck. Maybe even a dull headache.

Now is that any way to begin the rest of your life? Of course not! Trouble is, many of us are the slaves of certain subtle habits we don't even know we have. And those hidden habits could be the reason why the fabled sandman, who once sprinkled his soothing dust on you ever so lightly, may have lately taken to dropping 40-pound bags of Sakrete on your weary noggin, neck or spine.

Here are some things we can do about it.

1. Position Yourself for Relaxation

Usually we think of our muscles tightening up after excessive exertion, like a solid hour of shoveling snow. But you can get stiff doing nothing, too. If you have any tendency at all to backaches or arthritis, lying almost motionless in bed for eight hours can be more than enough to make you stiff from ankles to neck.

Here are some helpful tips from Henry Feffer, M.D., an orthopedic surgeon in Washington, D.C. First, if you have a tendency to wake up with backaches, try sleeping on your side with your legs curled up. Or else sleep on your back with a pillow under your knees. That flattens the part of your back that tends to sway in toward your stomach and takes some of the strain off the muscles. Try this just once and you may get to sleep faster just because it feels so good to have your legs supported by a pillow. Use a nice big fluffy one and put it right under your knees.

2. To Wake Up, Limber Up

During the time you are asleep, your body is in a kind of minihibernation. Your temperature actually goes down, and your circulation and breathing become sluggish. So take time to limber up before *getting* up, particularly if you wake up stiff. A mattress that doesn't support you well may be involved, but it's probably not as important as the fact that you've been motionless and in cold storage all those hours.

To ease out of the morning backache, one simple movement is to bring your knees up to your chest, lock your arms around your shins, hold for a few seconds and then lower your legs. Repeat several times. (On pages 4-6 is a somewhat more elaborate but very sensible little stretching routine given to us by the Kripalu Center for Holistic Health in Summit Station, Pennsylvania. One of our editors tried it and he says it makes him feel a lot better in the morning.)

3. Stiff? Try the Snugly Warm Approach

About five years ago, a doctor specializing in arthritis reported that the very bothersome morning stiffness sometimes associated with this disease could be much improved by spending the night cocooned inside a sleeping bag. During the ensuing years, we have heard from a number of *Prevention* magazine readers who found that this technique worked beautifully for them. One reader said that thermal underwear worked just as well and was easier to launder.

4. Customize Your Time in Bed

An especially good idea came from Wilse B. Webb, Ph.D., psychologist at the University of Florida in Gainesville. Dr. Webb told us the need for sleep varies greatly among individuals, with each person having his or her own specific requirements for sleep just as for nutrition. With nutrition, a person who functions best at a body weight of 150 pounds, let's say, can survive by adapting to a weight of 130. But he won't feel up to par; a certain vitality will be absent. The same goes for sleep requirements. The individual who needs nine hours of sleep may try to crowd all his sleep into seven hours, but he or she will have a continuous

(continued on page 6)

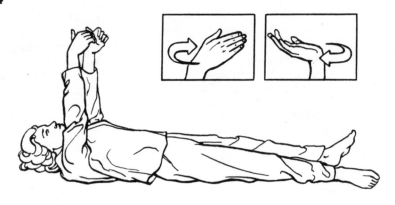

Remaining in bed or gently rising and lying on the floor beside the bed, lie on your back and slowly raise your arms vertically in the air. Rotate your wrists in each direction and gently lower.

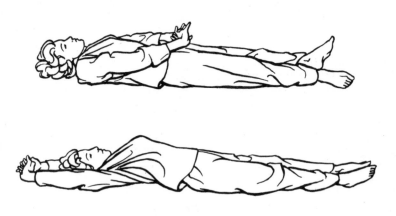

Clasp the hands on the stomach. Invert your palms so that they face your feet, and stretch them downward. Now slowly (all these movements should be done slowly) begin to lift them into the air, breathing in deeply and slowly and bringing them down to the floor behind or above your head, arms fully stretched out. Exhaling, stretch and arch your back, loosening your spine.

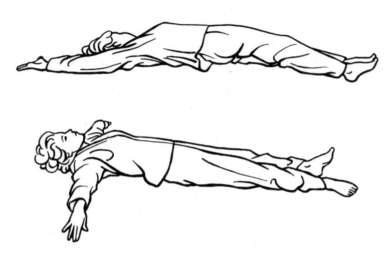

Unclasp your hands. Now, while inhaling, stretch your right arm and right leg in opposite directions so that they form a straight line, making the right side of your body longer than the left, while lifting the right hip. Now relax and exhale. Now do the left arm and leg. Stretch them fully, inhaling deeply while lifting and twisting the left hip. Exhale, slowly bringing your arms down, and totally extend them straight out from your body at shoulder height, touching the floor or bed. Relax for a moment, breathing deeply.

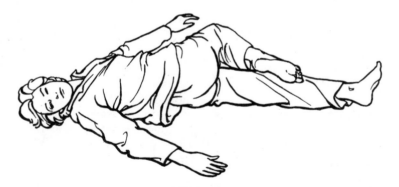

Inhaling, slowly raise your right knee, sliding the right foot along the ground until it is next to the left knee. Exhaling slowly, twist your body, bringing the right knee over toward the ground outside of your left thigh. As you do that, turn your head slowly to the right. Don't strain. Be very relaxed and enjoy the stretch. Now, exhaling, slowly go back to the center and slide the foot back to its starting position beside the other foot. Relax, then repeat with the other side.

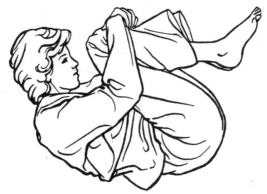

This exercise must be done on the floor, preferably on a thick, soft carpet. It is a more involved version of the simple exercise mentioned before, and very good for people who suffer from tight back muscles. First, gently come to a sitting position with your knees up to your chest and your feet on the floor. Your hands are clasped around your knees, your head bent forward. Now, begin to rock back onto your shoulders, keeping the spine well curved and the head tucked in so that your whole body is rolled up in a kind of ball. Rock backward and forward like this perhaps a dozen times, fairly briskly, so that the momentum helps keep you going. Breathe in as you rock back, and out as you rock forward. Then relax on your back.

struggle to wake up and will frequently feel fatigued—if not downright rotten.

Moral: A person who shortchanges himself on sleep may be cheating himself of his zest for living. Why cheat yourself of anything, let alone the enjoyment of life?

5. Learn to Fall Asleep Faster

Suppose you simply have trouble getting to sleep in the first place. Regrets about the past, tension in the present or anxiety about the future—these common aggravations can sometimes keep us up for hours. The next morning, you invariably wake up more weary than when you went to bed. And the rest of the day just drags.

Let's back up to the night before. Your body, as you lie there tossing and turning, is probably in a nightmarish state of biological turbulence. "Many poor sleepers are more aroused than good sleepers," writes sleep specialist Richard R. Bootzin, Ph.D., of Northwestern University, in a recent survey of sleep research. "Poor sleepers [have] higher rectal temperatures, higher skin resistance, more vasoconstrictions [narrowing of blood vessels] per minute and more body movements per hour than good sleepers." All of those symptoms mean that the insomniac's autonomic nervous system, which controls involuntary body functions, is preparing him perfectly for dodging rush-hour traffic—but not for sleep. If he can put his autonomic nervous system to sleep, the theory goes, the rest of him should follow (*Progress in Behavior Modification*, vol. 6, Academic Press, 1978).

For years, doctors casually prescribed sleeping pills for temporary insomnia. Many still do (to the tune of about 25 million prescriptions a year), but in the past three or four years, more and more physicians and psychologists are realizing that these drugs don't work and can be harmful if used frequently. A better way to send ourselves quickly to sleep, researchers are finding, is by learning simple skills—like muscle relaxation techniques, deep breathing, imagery, autogenic training and self-hypnosis—that can be applied when needed, without even leaving our beds.

RELAXATION. Progressive Relaxation is a particular form of muscle relaxation. Originated in the early 1900s by physiologist Edmund Jacobson, Progressive Relaxation or variations of it are still taught. One of these variations has been evaluated by Thomas D. Borkovec, Ph.D., a psychologist at Penn State University.

"We have the person start with the muscles of one hand, making a fist, holding it for seven seconds, and then relaxing it," says Dr. Borkovec, who teaches four-week and nine-week courses in relaxation.

"We ask the individual to learn to identify what both tension and relaxation feel like, so that he will be able to detect tension when trying to fall asleep. After sufficient practice, most people are able to deeply relax themselves within five minutes."

His students gradually learn to relax 16 of the body's muscle groups, Dr. Borkovec said. They also inhale when they tense their muscles, then exhale and relax very slowly (for about 45 seconds). That is good therapy for people whose main problem is falling asleep, and its effect improves with practice, Dr. Borkovec said. (See the chapter Lighten Up with Relaxation for detailed instruction on Progressive Relaxation.)

DEEP BREATHING. Proper breathing, just by itself, is another way to reassure the autonomic nervous system that it can tone down for the night. In one experiment in 1976, volunteers were asked to "focus passively on the physical sensations associated with their breathing and to repeat the mantra [a word or image to fix the mind on] 'in' and 'out' silently." Results indicated that this technique is as effective as Progressive Relaxation (*Progress in Behavior Modification,* vol. 6, Academic Press, 1978).

The fine points of breathing have been described by psychologist Beata Jencks, Ph.D., in her book, *Your Body: Biofeedback at Its Best* (Nelson-Hall, 1977).

"Imagine inhaling through your fingertips," Dr. Jencks writes, "up the arms, into the shoulders, and then exhaling down the trunk into the abdomen and legs, and leisurely out at the toes. Repeat, and feel how this slow, deep breathing [called the Long Breath] affects the whole body, the abdomen, the flanks and the chest. Do not move the shoulders while doing the Long Breath."

To inhale deeply, Dr. Jencks advises, pretend to inhale the fragrance of the first flower in spring, or imagine that your breathing rises and falls like ocean waves, or that the surface area of your lungs—if laid out flat—would cover a tennis court. That's how much air you can feel yourself breathing in.

IMAGERY. Imagery can accompany breathing exercises, and your choice of images doesn't have to be limited to the traditional sheep leaping over a split-rail fence. Any image that you personally associate with feelings of peace or contentment will work well.

One sleep researcher, Quentin Regestein, M.D., director of the Sleep Clinic at Brigham and Women's Hospital in Boston, told us that one of his patients imagines a huge sculpture of the numeral 1, hewn out of marble, with ivy growing over it, surrounded by a pleasant rural landscape. Then she goes on to the numeral 2, and adds further embellishment, such as cherubs hovering above the numeral. "She tells me that she usually falls asleep before she reaches 50," Dr. Regestein said.

"Insomniacs come here from all over the world," he continued, "and ask me to prescribe a sleep cure for them. They are sometimes surprised to find that careful scientific investigation substantiates that commonsense remedies really work."

SELF-SUGGESTION. Autogenic training is another natural and potent sleep aid. This technique acts on the premise that your mind can compel your body to relax by concentrating on feelings of heaviness and warmth. Through mental suggestion, the "heavy" muscles actually do relax, and the "warm" flesh receives better circulation, resulting in "a state of low physiological arousal," said Dr. Bootzin.

In an experiment in 1968, researchers taught 16 college-student insomniacs to focus their attention on warmth and heaviness. At the end of the experiment, the students had cut down their average time needed to fall asleep from 52 to 22 minutes (*Journal of Abnormal Psychology,* June, 1968). These results matched the findings made by Dr. Bootzin in the Chicago area in 1974: "Daily practice of either Progressive Relaxation or autogenic training produced 50 percent improvement in time to fall asleep by the end of the one-month treatment period" (*Journal of Abnormal Psychology,* June, 1974).

A Raggedy Ann doll, says Dr. Jencks, is one image that can facilitate autogenic training. To feel heavy, she says, "make yourself comfortable and allow your eyes to close. Then lift one arm a little and let it drop. Let it drop heavily, as if it were the arm of one of those floppy dolls or animals. Choose one in your imagination. Choose a doll, or an old beloved, soft teddy bear." Once the mind fixes on the doll's image, Dr. Jencks says, lifting and dropping the arm in your imagination works as well as really letting it drop.

To invoke feelings of warmth, Dr. Jencks adds, "Imagine that you put your rag doll into the sun. Let it be warmed by the sun. . . . You are the giant rag doll, and you are lying in the sun; all your limbs are nice and warm, but your head is lying in the shade and is comfortably cool."

Self-hypnosis, though it may require some practice in advance, has also been shown to help people fall asleep. Researchers in England compared the sleep-inducing ability of sleeping pills, self-hypnosis and a placebo (dummy pill) on 18 volunteer insomniacs. Some of the volunteers learned to put themselves into a trance by picturing themselves in a "warm, safe place—possibly on a holiday someplace pleasant."

When they had put themselves into a trance, the researchers told them, they would be able to give themselves the suggestions "that this would pass into a deep, refreshing sleep, waking up at the usual time in the morning, feeling wide awake."

The results showed that the subjects fell asleep faster by hypnotizing themselves than by using either the drug or the placebo. None of the self-hypnotized sleepers needed an hour to fall asleep, while three in the placebo group and four in the drug group did. Twelve in the self-hypnotized group fell asleep in less than 30 minutes, while only seven and ten, respectively, in the other groups did (*Journal of the Royal Society of Medicine,* October, 1979).

6. When It Comes to Sleeping, Be a Creature of Habit

If none of the above techniques seem to work for you, there are several changes in daily habits that can, with practice, help you to fall asleep a lot faster in the future.

■ Go to sleep and wake up at regular hours. Monte Stahl, associate director of the Sleep Disorder Center at Presbyterian Hospital in Oklahoma City, Oklahoma, told us that "an irregular bedtime is disruptive to good sleep." So try to find a time at which you are naturally and pretty consistently tired. Then hit the hay with just as much promptness as you wake up.

Other hints that many sleep researchers recommend:

■ Go to bed only when sleepy.

■ Don't nap during the day.

■ Use your bed only for sleeping and sex; don't read, eat or watch TV in bed.

■ Keep your bedroom fairly cool.

Rituals also play a role in falling asleep. Dr. Regestein told us that when dogs go to sleep, they always sniff around for a warm and comfortable spot, circle it, and finally coil up in their favorite sleeping position. People are a bit like that, he said. They fall asleep most easily when they proceed through a nightly ritual — flossing their teeth, for example, and then curling into their favorite sleeping position. In support of that theory, researchers in 1930 found that children who assumed a particular posture when going to bed fell asleep faster.

7. Exercise Increases the Quality of Your Sleep

Most of us know that a good bout of exercise during the day makes it easier to fall asleep at night. But did you know that when you exercise, the quality of the sleep you get changes for the better? It's true. What happens is that the rhythm of your sleep changes so you spend relatively more time in a phase that sleep researchers call slow-wave sleep, or SWS. Slow-wave sleep is a very deep form of sleep which is also the most restorative, especially to the physical body. Samuel Dunkell, M.D., a New York psychoanalyst and author of the book *Sleep Positions* (William Morrow, 1977), told us that "strenuous exercise for half an hour three times a week increases SWS. But this should not be done too close to sleep, because after strenuous exercise, the body is very stimulated. Several hours before bedtime is fine."

Arthur J. Spielman, Ph.D., a clinical psychologist specializing in sleep disorders, added that exercise done in the morning has no effect on slow-wave sleep that night. So it looks like the best time to exercise — at least as far as sleeping goes — would be, for most people, between about 4 P.M. and 8 P.M.

But here is the really interesting thing. The exercise-for-better-sleep routine works much better in people who are physically fit. Research by an Australian scientist reported in 1978 revealed that when fit and unfit people were given exercise, the amount of slow-wave sleep increased in the fit people, but not in those who weren't. Curiously, the fit people had relatively more slow-wave sleep even on days when they weren't exercising. That indicates, perhaps, that their bodies have become conditioned to restoring themselves more effectively.

Don't think that exercise won't do you any good, though, just because you aren't fit. All it takes is a good solid half hour of rapid walking in the evening every day for a few weeks, and you'll be getting the benefits of SWS along with all the others that come with regular exercise. (See the next chapter, Energize with Exercise, for more on the invigorating powers of physical activity.)

HOW SOME OF US WAKE UP

Do you rely on an eye-opening cup of coffee to get yourself going in the morning, only to lapse back toward lethargy a little later when the effects of the brew wear off? Here's how some people sidestep coffee and *really* get mobilized in the morning.

Maggie Kuhn, founder of the Gray Panthers, a national activist organization against age discrimination, based in Philadelphia: "I'm basically a night person. To wake up in the morning I do mild stretching exercises and take a warm bath. I have arthritis and it helps to soak for a while. It's refreshing and relaxing. And the exercises help loosen the stiffness." Maggie also believes that it helps you get going in the morning if you have goals that "go beyond your own self-interests. Having a purpose is so important. It keeps me young."

Lawrence Welk: According to his personal secretary, Laurie Rector, "Mr. Welk survives on very little sleep indeed—11:00 P.M. to 4:30 A.M. After getting up, he goes for a swim, shoots some golf balls, and is in his office at 7:00 A.M. He can fall asleep instantly, anywhere, and wake up raring to go. He takes a short afternoon nap."

Robert A. Butler, Ph.D., chairman of the department of behavioral sciences at the University of Chicago: "I don't wake up feeling fresh in the morning. So I try to run four to eight miles before breakfast. That gets me going. When I don't run, I don't feel as sharp. I'm not saying it would work for everyone, but it works for me."

Eileen Ford, vice president of the Ford Modeling Agency,
(continued)

New York City: "I wake up feeling great since I gave up drinking. I learned I can have a good time at a party without drinking. Wine was the worst of all. It would make me sleepy, and I'd sleep for about three hours, but then I would wake up and that would be that. The first thing I do in the morning is vigorous deep breathing exercises. Then I exercise in place, jogging on a foam rubber jogging board for about five minutes. And each night, before going to bed, I take two oyster-shell calcium pills."

Lenore Hershey, editor in chief of Ladies' Home Journal *in New York City:* "I go to bed early and try not to watch anything that's too disturbing (like the news) right before bedtime. I try to get some physical exercise each day, even if it's only walking, to help me feel less tired. I don't eat or drink anything after dinner since I think that keeps me awake. If I can't sleep, I take a warm bath. I think of some soothing, memorable occasions, maybe even from 20 years before. I do suffer from insomnia sometimes. I have learned that the best way to handle it is not to fight it. When I can't sleep, I will stay in bed and let my mind do something constructive. I usually wake up feeling refreshed in the morning."

For more information on exercise and stretching as wake-up activities, see the next chapter, Energize with Exercise.

Energize with Exercise

CHAPTER 2

When you hear of Olympic athletes setting new world records time after time, you may find yourself wondering just what the limits of human energy and endurance may be—especially when *you* get winded just vacuuming the dining room rug or running to catch a cab. *How do they do it?* you may ask.

Gradually. After all, no one was born running the 100-yard dash. On the other hand, those athletes didn't get in such great shape by watching TV night after night, either. Their energy and stamina comes from a source available to each and every one of us: regular doses of vitamin X—exercise, that is.

One of the comments we hear most frequently, especially from the housekeeper of the family, is, "You mean to say that with all the housework and laundry I do, I still need to exercise?" And the answer is yes. Because what we're talking about is not mere movement, but the kind of activity that gets your heart rate and respiration humming along at a healthy clip for 15 to 30 minutes at least three times a week. A brisk walk, running, swimming, cycling, gardening, hiking, dancing—anything that uses the large muscles of the legs and gets the blood pumping through the heart, lungs and the rest of the body.

Exercise? When I feel tired to begin with? Wouldn't sleep be better?

Not always. If you're behind on your rest—or put in an especially long, hard day—then sleep may be just what you need. But if what you feel is just the routine accumulation of tension and restlessness, exercise is the answer.

13

Exercise Rewinds Your Body Clock

Exercise energizes in two ways. First, exercise increases your ability to handle more of a work load. At the same time, an evening run, for example, or a brisk walk around the block, can relieve accumulated muscle tension, giving you a second wind for the closing hours of the day. What you think is fatigue may really be your body's way of crying out for stimulation.

But exercise is just for kids, you might say. *Or athletes. But not this old body.* The truth is, though, exercise is *not* just kids' stuff. What's more, evidence shows that exercise not only peps you up, but also helps keep you young—physically *and* mentally.

Activity Keeps You Young

According to Walter M. Bortz II, M.D., of the Palo Alto Medical Clinic in California, aging people show the same metabolic breakdown as people subjected to forced inactivity. Which means, logically, that exercise should slow aging.

Maximal oxygen volume, Dr. Bortz told the annual meeting of the American Geriatrics Society in April, 1979, decreases about 1 percent every year with age and lack of exercise. That means that every part of the body of an inactive older person is getting less and less cell-nourishing oxygen the older he grows. However, if such a person refuses to take that sitting down, he or she can defy the aging process. According to Dr. Bortz, with moderate exercise an older person can achieve the maximal oxygen volume of a person 15 years younger. A very active older person can achieve the maximal oxygen volume of a person 40 years younger. And besides increasing oxygen intake, exercise can compensate for bodily decline by increasing heart output, lung capacity and blood volume.

Exercise may also help keep our reflexes quick. All too often, reflexes (which scientists measure by testing reaction time, the time between a stimulus and its reaction) slow down as a person gets older. But that may not always be the case. In a study of reaction time and aging, researchers at the department of physical education at San Diego University tested 64 men and women ranging from 23 to 59 years of age. Half of the volunteers were runners; the other half, sedentary people. The researchers measured their reaction time by having them move their hands when a light flashed. The results showed that reaction time does indeed decline with age—except in people who exercise. Their reactions were just as quick as those of the younger people in the study.

Exercise Pulls Pounds off Your Back

How many energetic fat people can you name? Hardly any, we'd wager. Being overweight is like trying to get through the day with a 15-pound (or 20- or 30-pound) sack of potatoes strapped to your back. And when you think about it, the first thing a mountain climber does when he stops to rest is take the pack off his back. But if you're overweight, you're forced to carry your pack around all day and all night. No wonder every movement is a chore.

If we've been a little blunt here, it's only to impress upon you what a difference those extra pounds can make on your energy levels. And it's not only physical weight you're carrying around—overweight is also a psychological burden. Remember how Dracula shunned mirrors? Well, so do fat people—but for different reasons. While vampires don't reflect in mirrors, fat people wish they didn't. Their self-image is often that poor. Inside, they may dread getting out and being seen. So if you lose those extra pounds, not only do you shed your physical burden, but your self-esteem goes up—and so does your desire to get out and up and *do* things.

Exercise is one sure way, along with a little sensible dieting, to lighten up. Combined with the suggestions in Part 2, Supernutrition for Work and Play, exercise can go a long way toward boosting your pep quotient.

Exercise for Mental Pep

You don't have to have a weight problem for exercise to give you a psychological lift. Studies on the attitudes of elderly people show that those who exercise feel better about themselves than those who don't. On a psychological test designed to measure a person's self-image, people who exercised the least felt that they didn't live up to their ideal image of themselves. Those who exercised the most showed a good body image, close to their desired image of themselves (*Medicine and Science in Sports,* vol. 8, no. 4, 1976).

It follows from this that taking up a program of exercise can change personality for the better. "We know now that personality in adults is a dynamic thing, not a static thing," said A. H. Ismail, professor of physical education at Purdue University (and former Olympic basketball player). "There can be changes, and the changes that are produced through a fitness regimen are in a positive direction." For 20 years, Dr. Ismail has been conducting fitness programs involving hundreds of participants and has found that nonexercisers who scored low on emotional stability tests showed marked improvement after completing a fitness program.

Exercise has been shown to improve not only the self-image and psychological strength of people, but also their mental sharpness.

It stands to reason that good oxygen levels in the blood can boost brain power. Working with that logical hunch, Claude Fell Merzbacher, Ph.D., of the department of natural science at San Diego State University, gathered together a group of 31 volunteers to test the effect of diet and exercise on their mental skills. The volunteers were part of a group enrolled in a diet, exercise and education program at the Longevity Research Institute of Santa Monica. The average age of the group was 60 years, and every member suffered from cardiovascular disease or some other degenerative disease such as diabetes, claudication (a circulatory problem) or arthritis—diseases that at an advanced age are especially trying and distracting. For 26 days the volunteers followed the Institute's exercise program, which consisted mostly of daily walks.

At the same time, the group ate a wholesome high-fiber diet containing no fats or oils except those in grains, vegetables and fruits, and very small amounts of meat, minimal cholesterol, no simple carbohydrates, especially refined sugar, honey and molasses, and no added salt.

Both before and after the completion of the regimen, the group was given various tests. On one test, which measured socialization, self-control, tolerance, achievement and intellectual efficiency, volunteers who took it showed higher scores after the regimen. This meant improved verbal fluency, quick, clear thinking, intellectual efficiency and perceptiveness.

On another test, which measured changes in mental sharpness, the group again scored higher after the combined diet and exercise regimen. And all this in the remarkably short time of less than a month (*Perceptual and Motor Skills,* April, 1979).

Exercise can rejuvenate your body and sharpen your mind. But "perhaps the greatest benefit of maintaining physical fitness is the degree of independence it affords." suggested C. Carson Conrad, executive director of the President's Council on Physical Fitness and Sports. "This is a quality to be prized in the later years of life. There is a great psychological and financial advantage in having the ability to plan and do things without depending on relatives, friends or hired help. To drive your own car, to succeed with do-it-yourself projects rather than trying to find and pay someone else for the service, and to go and come as you please in terms of physical ability to do so—these are major assets that we believe regular physical exercise can help achieve."

No matter what your age, then, exercise will keep you going.

"People who exercise regularly report that they feel better, have more energy, often require less sleep," states the report *Healthy People—The Surgeon General's Report on Health Promotion and Disease Prevention,* published in 1979 by the U.S. Department of Health, Education and Welfare. Aside from losing weight, says the report, regular exercisers improve muscular strength and flexibility. In turn many also experience psychological benefits, including enhanced self-esteem, greater self-reliance, decreased anxiety, and relief from mild depression.

A Brisk Walk Will Do It

You needn't be a runner to grow young and quick through exercise. "A good brisk walk will do the trick for the vast majority of people," said Henry J. Ralston, Ph.D., from the department of anatomy at the University of California Medical Center at San Francisco.

There's a right way to walk if your aim is to give yourself a lift. First, be sure to wear a comfortable pair of shoes or sneakers. As you move, breathe very deeply and allow your entire body to gracefully be involved in the activity. Be sure to walk vigorously—at least for a short while—so that you stimulate your heart and circulatory system to function more completely and effectively. Do not strain and do not try to race. Instead walk as long as is gently comfortable for you and then rest.

When a person can walk three miles in 45 minutes, he is ready for jogging (if he wants to make the switch). But don't start with jogging right off. Try 20 steps of jogging, then walk until rested, then jog 20 steps again. After a few weeks, you'll be ready to jog nonstop.

If a pool is available, you might swim several days each week. As with brisk walking, you do not want to race or strain but instead use the vigorous swimming motion as a way to limber up your whole body and stimulate your heart. Breathe deeply and include your whole body in the activity. Be certain to relax and rest after you are done.

The important step, the "biggest change," according to William L. Haskell, Ph.D., assistant professor of cardiology at Stanford University School of Medicine, "is to get the people who are doing nothing to do something." Besides brisk walking, running, stair climbing, cycling, gardening and home repairs are some activities he suggests. Dancing is also rejuvenating. All those are excellent activities for strengthening the body and releasing stress and tension. Such vigorous activities are especially helpful in improving cardiovascular and respiratory functioning and go a long way to vitalize the heart and lungs while relieving general fatigue and the kind of chronic drowsiness that often accompanies sedentary life and work styles.

Start Slow

You've probably heard the saying, "You have to walk before you can run." Well, it's true.

Don't expect to jump into a vigorous exercise program. Start slow. Warm up. Old hearts especially need to be worked slowly at first. Each day do just a little more. Start with modified calisthenics, then add one more step each time you exercise. The only competition is with yourself, progressively improving strength, flexibility and endurance.

A reasonable goal for any individual ought to be 15 to 30 minutes of exercise at least three times a week. Beginners should start slowly, and people over 40 should be examined by a physician first.

The question arises as to how much exercise an older person can do without its being too dangerous. According to Don S. Wenger, M.D., president of the National Association for Human Development (NAHD), our bodies have a wonderful set of sensors that warn of stress. Marked shortness of breath, severe joint pain and chest pain are symptoms to watch for. As soon as you feel bothered, stop and rest. "If it squeaks, you need it. If it hurts, stop!" is a good way to check your limitations.

Older people are just as trainable as younger ones, emphasized Herbert deVries, Ph.D., director of the exercise physiology laboratory, Andrus Gerontology Center, University of Southern California. They can become active even if they have never been in good shape or previously active in their lives. "We were all amazed at how well older men and women swam after six months of instruction in an experimental program. Some 80-year-olds could swim the crawl 20 to 30 widths of the pool. That is better than many college kids can do."

People often think it's their due to be able to slow down and have others wait on them. Sure it's fun to be pampered, but you can be pampered to death. Many of our laborsaving devices are doing just that! With power mowers, snow blowers and other power tools, we are losing much of our forced activity. Apartments no longer have gardens to dig in or repairs to be made. A steady program of exercise is the only answer.

It has been proven that active people lead much better lives. Body rebuilding must constantly go on. The building materials are a sensible diet with regular physical and mental activity. To quote Dr. Wenger, "Use the brain, use the body, use the life—don't lose it!"

Turn Your Home into an Energy Center

We have spaces in our houses and apartments for all major functions of life. A kitchen is provided for cooking, a dining area for eating, bathrooms for washing and elimination, bedrooms for sleeping and a living room for resting and socializing. Some people go beyond those basic components of shelter and also have rooms for their hobbies, watching TV, washing clothes, protecting their cars, and doing business at home.

Robert Rodale, *Prevention* magazine's editor, explained how he converted unused space in his home to a family "energy center."

"We have a finished basement, intended to be a game room and place for parties. When our children were younger they used it as a playroom. But our older children grew up and moved out, so the room was unused most of the time.

"Two years ago, I began making it into an exercise room. First, we got an exercise bicycle and put it in front of the TV set in the basement. Pedaling while watching a program makes indoor exercise easier. Then I got an indoor jogger, a kind of minitrampoline. My youngest son saw what was happening and moved his weight-training barbells into the room. Later I added a unique cross-country ski machine, which provides a fine workout of both legs and upper body without stressing the joints.

"Putting these devices in one room created what might be called motivational chemistry. We now find that exercising indoors is more fun, especially when several people are in the room together. We switch from one activity to another, and keep each other company. Of course, the room is used most in the winter, when outdoor exercise is discouraged by bad weather. Actually, I find that I am in better shape in spring after a winter of indoor exercise than I am in the fall.

"The cost of setting up that room was low, especially since we used space that was going to waste. And if you use some imagination, you can set up a minigym for even less money. A jump rope is a good motivator, and costs hardly anything. Putting an inexpensive mat on the floor lets you do yoga and flexibility exercises."

If you can't spare the space in your house, you might consider joining the local YMCA, YWCA, a spa, or other physical activity center for exercises like swimming, dancing, racquetball or tennis. But remember, some of the best exercises—walking, gardening, hiking, and running—require very little in the way of special equipment or surroundings.

How to Make Time for Exercise

Regular exercise does not necessarily mean *daily* exercise. Michael L. Pollock, Ph.D., of Mount Sinai Medical Center in Milwaukee, says that exercising three days a week seems to be a good compromise. Once or twice a week is not enough to maintain physical gains. Three days a week comes close to maximizing both cardiovascular fitness and weight control, two major health benefits of exercise. People who exercise five times a week obtain some additional improvement, but probably not enough to justify the threefold increased risk of injury. "Unless you are a competitive athlete, or sincerely enjoy what you are doing," said Dr. Pollock, "you do not need to exercise more than every other day."

But where do I find the time? some ask.

You do not find the time. You *make* the time. Many people have an exaggerated idea of the time it takes to exercise, but it only takes about 30 minutes. Morning people may find they enjoy a run before breakfast. An evening person may look forward to a brisk walk or bicycle ride before nightfall.

If you have trouble squeezing a half hour out of the day for yourself, perhaps your day is not organized very well. Take inventory of your time. Maybe you can skip some TV, or ask someone in the family to help with dinner a few nights. Or eat a little later. Or take a long lunch hour and make up the time in the morning. Or get up and jog in place for 15 minutes instead of your midmorning and midafternoon coffee breaks. Chances are, there is someplace during the day when 30 minutes can be found.

Stretching — The Other Side of Exercise

Most of the activities we regard as exercise primarily involve muscle contraction. The muscles manipulated in most sports are repeatedly tensed up, pulled shorter, by the movement. That's exactly what you have to do to muscles if your intent is to make them stronger.

But if you want to maintain the muscle flexibility you need, not just to run marathons, but to stay active and comfortable into your later years, you have to *stretch* muscles as well as contract them. Most people are not even aware how flexible their joints can be, because their muscles are not loose enough to allow them the fullest possible range of movement.

Joint stiffness, an affliction common to aging, is probably

more a problem of muscles and connective tissues than of the joints themselves. Experiments at Johns Hopkins Medical School with the wrists of cats found that the most important factors in flexibility are the muscles, the tendons and the capsule of tissue enclosing the joint. The scientists found that the friction generated by the rubbing at the joint itself was a minor factor limiting movement of the wrist. That was true even in joints afflicted with arthritis (*Journal of Applied Physiology,* vol. 17, 1962).

Now how can you expect to feel fit and frisky with stiff joints? You can't. Weakness or stiffness of muscles is a problem that can make anyone feel his age. "Too much tension and too little exercise greatly increase the natural loss of muscular fitness with age," writes Hans Kraus, M.D., former associate professor at the Institute of Rehabilitation Medicine, New York University. To help older people with back pain and other muscle problems, Dr. Kraus developed a YMCA exercise program stressing relaxation, stretching of tight muscles and strengthening of weak ones. This program is now offered in nearly 1,000 YMCAs around the country and has an 80 percent rate of success.

"Reconditioning these patients," writes Dr. Kraus, "simply means reclaiming abilities that never should have been lost" (*Geriatrics,* June, 1978). So to increase the flexibility of the joints, you have to work mainly with the muscles and connective tissue. Pliable muscles, tendons and ligaments would make for flexible joints.

But ligaments, the tissues that hold bones together, and tendons, which attach muscles to bones, are both inflexible, inelastic tissues. A ligament or tendon stretched beyond its rather meager limits will not return to its original length. It doesn't bounce back as it should. The joint it holds together becomes too loose, and prone to injury.

That leaves the muscles. Muscles are much more elastic than tendons and ligaments. A muscle repeatedly and properly stretched continues to bounce back, but it bounces back to a longer resting shape. Since the muscle is meant to move the frame, rather than hold it together, this is all for the good. A properly stretched set of muscles means maximum freedom of movement.

Stretch Gently; Don't Bounce

Many people think that they're stretching their muscles when they go through bouncy, calisthenic exercises like touching their toes. You bounce down quickly to touch your toes, then pop back up into a standing position. But that bounce is what causes problems. Whenever a muscle is stretched too quickly or with too much force, the splinting reflex is set off. That's a protective mechanism wherein the muscle stiffens, forming a natural, rigid splint—comparable to a splint applied to a broken leg.

You meet the same kind of resistance when you stretch in a standing position. Muscles in your legs hold your body up by contracting. Stretching leg muscles in a standing position is not as effective as stretching while lying down or sitting, because you're again working against contracted muscles.

Ben E. Benjamin, Ph.D., author of the book *Sports Without Pain* (Summit, 1979), emphasizes that the best way to stretch is to ease yourself into the stretch position. Stretching is a gentle, conditioning exercise. Relaxation is very important. Once you have extended your muscles as far as they want to go, don't force them any farther. Just keep breathing normally and hold the position for 10 to 15 seconds. Next time you might stretch farther, and hold the position longer.

"You must be able to tell where the action is happening," Dr. Benjamin writes. "Pay attention to precisely where the pulling sensation is. You should feel the pull in the meaty part of the muscle. If the sensation is felt near a joint only, you are stretching the ligament or tendon. Always try to do the exercise so that you feel it throughout the bulk of the muscle."

Dr. Benjamin says that the best time to stretch is after a warmup. Warm muscles, surging with blood, are more pliable than cold. A common mistake, Dr. Benjamin told us, is that "people confuse warming up with stretching. They do stretching exercises to warm up when they should be doing it the other way around. Stretching is not really a good way to warm up. It's good for cooling down after exercise." Both Dr. Benjamin and Dr. deVries recommend that stretching be done at the end of an exercise routine.

Seven Big Stretches for Renewed Energy

The muscles that probably need the most stretching are those in the lower part of the body. Muscles in the legs and lower back are almost constantly in use during the day, holding us erect. Because of that constant contraction, they are more susceptible to shortening and tightness. We have picked the exercises on pages 24-27 because they generally stretch those lower-body muscles, and because they can be done with relative ease, even in your office after a midday workout.

TAKE A "STRETCH BREAK" INSTEAD OF A COFFEE BREAK

Shoulders aching and tired because you've been desk-bound for hours? Or maybe you're just feeling lazy for lack of activity. To get your body humming again, try these abbreviated stretching techniques:

■ Stand erect with your arms behind your back, hands lightly clasped together. Slowly bend forward. At the same time slowly bring the arms behind you backward and up, until they are pointing directly overhead, or as near as can be done without force. This refreshing exercise takes only a moment but makes you feel as though you had a long rest. In addition, when practiced several times daily, it is a great help in maintaining more erect posture.

■ The circle is another exercise swing that stretches and stimulates your whole body. It's a great wake-up exercise and a wonderful invigorator during the day. Stand upright and bring lightly clasped hands over the head, centering the head between the arms.

Breathing deeply, bend the body sideways to the right, keeping the head centered between the arms. Continue to move slowly to the right, then forward toward the floor. Continue in a sweeping motion without interruption to the left and on up until you are in an upright position. Repeat in the opposite direction.

■ Get into the habit of pacing. Instead of dropping into a chair to mull over a problem, get up and move around. As a general rule, never sit for more than an hour and a half without standing, stretching and walking or pacing for at least five minutes. You'll go back to what you were doing refreshed, and you'll be more efficient at it.

■ One of our favorite upright "stretchers" is walking in place through a doorway with the arms stretched overhead and the fingers touching the top of the archway. This is marvelously stimulating, for it pulls everything from the ankles right up to the rib cage and shoulders. Even the neck receives a beneficial massage, for you can feel the pull and surge. Try it and feel the exhilaration. It is also an excellent way to help overcome tension.

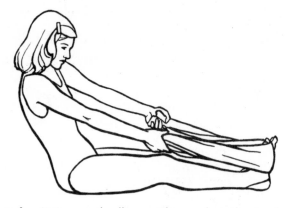

Calf Stretch—*Sitting on the floor, with your feet about a foot apart, place a towel around the ball of your foot. Without locking your knee, but holding it straight and steady, pull the towel toward you by leaning back. When you feel the stretch in the calf muscle, hold it for about 15 seconds. If it hurts, let up, or don't hold it as long. Alternate feet for two to four stretches. Gradually work up to 30-second stretches.*

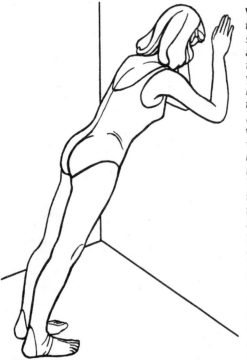

Wall Lean—*Move on to the wall lean for further stretching of the calves after you have mastered the towel stretch. With your feet two to three inches apart, stand three to five feet from the wall. Put your hands on the wall directly in front of you and bend your elbows until your forearms are resting against the wall. Your feet should be positioned as far as possible from the wall with your heels on the floor and your legs straight. After holding the position for 10 to 15 seconds, walk toward the wall and relax. The wall lean is fairly tough, so repeat it only three or four times. Over time you may build up to stretches as long as a minute.*

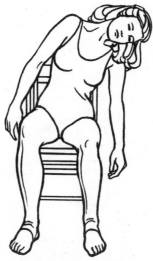

Side Stretch—*Sit in a chair with your feet about a foot apart, and bend your body to the right, imagining as you do so that you are lifting upward against the bend. Don't hold this stretch, just repeat on the left side, then go back to the right. Bend five times on each side. As the stretch becomes easier, add more weight to it by holding your hands behind your head as you bend. For even more weight later on, hold your hands up above your head as you bend.*

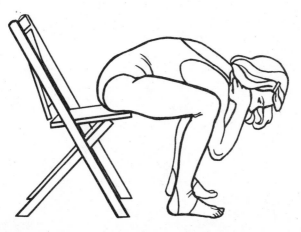

Back Stretch—*Sit in the same position in an armless chair. Bend forward, bringing your arms and shoulders between your knees. Lean forward as if you were going to put your elbows on the floor. Repeat the stretch several times, and gradually build up your holding time.*

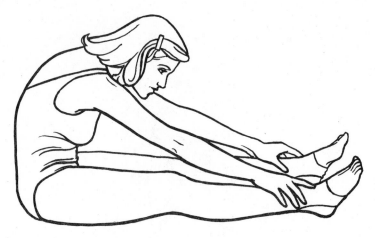

Bath Stretch—One relaxing way to stretch tired legs is in a bathtub full of warm water. Sitting in the tub with your legs straight, bend forward slowly until you feel the stretch in the muscles at the back of your legs. Relax, keep breathing normally, and hold the stretch for at least 50 or 60 seconds.

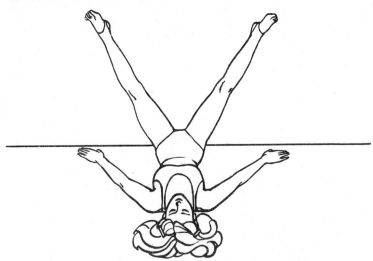

Inner Thigh Stretch—For this stretch, you need an empty wall about six feet wide. Lie on your back with your legs stretched against the wall, at a 90-degree angle to your body. Your buttocks and heels should be touching the wall. With your knees slightly bent, open your legs as far as they will go. Let gravity do most of the work of pulling your legs down. Hold that position as long as you feel comfortable, up to five minutes at a time.

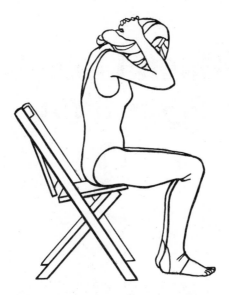

Neck Stretch—*While either sitting or standing, clasp your hands behind your neck and let your head fall forward. Hold that position for 10 to 15 seconds, then raise your head and rest. Repeat the stretch, only this time hold your hands an inch higher at the base of your skull. That is the maximum stretch, and should be done only if it is comfortable.*

Lighten Up with Relaxation

CHAPTER 3

How often do you start your day feeling fresh and fit, only to end up tense and tired before the morning is over?

For many of us, that fatigue is a direct result of stress in our lives. And sometimes it's just one stress after another. A vending machine that steals our quarters. Or financial concerns. Or back-to-back deadlines. Or problems raising the children. *Any* added demands on our personal energy can wear us out. Even the stress of *enjoying* life. Some people, in fact, have so much drive that they forget to give their bodies a break now and then.

But even though stress affects all of us, many people aren't aware of how it slowly saps their natural vitality. If unreleased, all that "residual tension" (as stress is sometimes called) makes us pushovers for fatigue. You see, going around wired up all day is *work*. It wastes energy, like a car with its idle set too high. So it's no wonder that stress makes so many of us poop out at midday, or come home at night barely able to do much more than stare at the TV tube.

And yet, more sleep is not necessarily the answer. Who wants to doze their life away when there are sights to see, good times to be enjoyed, so many things we'd like to do? *Relaxation* is the better solution.

To deal with the effects of stress, there are natural and effective ways to relax that leave us *rested yet alert*. "In recent years it has been demonstrated in the laboratory that actual sleep is not necessary to relieve fatigue provided the rest period is characterized by total relaxation and total concentration on pleasant, stimulating, constructive thoughts," wrote M. F. Graham,

28

M.D., a physician with a special interest in physical fitness and author of *Inner Energy: How to Overcome Fatigue* (Sterling, 1979). Other researchers and health professionals have arrived at the same conclusion.

We'd like to share some of their methods of relaxation with you. Choose one or two that best suit your disposition and routine. Then practice daily for best results. Learning to relax is much like learning a new sport or musical instrument: it's largely a matter of regular practice. After just a few practice sessions, you'll be able to use your new skill whenever you begin to feel dragged down by the whirligig of life.

The Relaxation Response

A technique called the Relaxation Response, which slows the pulse and rate of breathing, takes five minutes to learn and is sometimes also known as meditation. But before we pass along the technique, we want to point out that "meditation" in this sense does not mean thinking profound thoughts about the nature of the universe or anything like that. In fact, it means thinking about nothing, nothing at all. Random thoughts are bound to pop into our heads no matter what we do, but total freedom from extraneous thoughts is not required in meditation. The idea is to prevent the *continuity* of thought: that is, dwelling on one idea and considering its implications. During this relaxation technique, you allow thoughts and negative emotions such as anxiety to simply pass by.

The technique for eliciting the Relaxation Response was developed by Herbert Benson, M.D., of Harvard Medical School and director of the Hypertension Section of Boston's Beth Israel Hospital, who has been working with relaxation techniques for over ten years. Dr. Benson and others have shown in clinical studies that meditating for 10 to 20 minutes twice a day can be remarkably effective not only in improving total health and well-being, but also in reducing high blood pressure, of which stress is a strong cofactor. He believes that it's a temporary slowdown of bodily processes, repeated twice a day, that's responsible for the improved health of the "relaxers" he has observed.

All the different meditative practices of both Eastern and Western cultural traditions, he says, have been grounded in four basic components which are needed to evoke the Relaxation Response in the body.

The first is a quiet environment free of distractions. A quiet room is suitable, or a place of worship. The second requirement is a mental device, a word or object you can keep in your mind, much like the dangling watch used by movie hypnotists. The trick is to focus all your attention on the mental device—for example, by repeating the same word over and over to yourself.

The third requirement flows from focus on such a device. You need to assume a passive attitude. Distracting thoughts are simply disregarded, and you redirect your attention to the mental device. You do not worry about how well you are performing the technique. The object is to relax, after all. The fourth requirement is simply to assume a comfortable position, so that there is no distracting muscle tension.

The Relaxation Response is remarkably simple to learn. First, select a quiet room and sit in a comfortable chair. Adjust yourself so that you are as relaxed as possible. That will probably mean slouching forward a bit, resting your hands on your thighs, and keeping your feet flat on the floor, somewhat in front of the position of your knees.

Close your eyes. Now consciously relax all your muscles, beginning with your feet. Move up through your legs, your stomach, your chest, your arms, your neck, and even your face, jaws and mouth. When your jaw muscles are really relaxed, your lower teeth will probably not be touching your uppers.

Breathe through your nose, and draw the breath into your belly, which should be rising and falling. Become aware of your breathing, but don't make a big deal out of taking deep breaths. They aren't necessary. Breathe normally and naturally.

Now, as you breathe out, silently say the word "one" to yourself. Inhale. Exhale and again repeat the word "one."

Keep the muscles of your body relaxed and continue breathing rhythmically and easily in and out, repeating the "one" with every exhalation.

As we said, it's only natural that stray thoughts are going to pop into your head. Don't worry about them; they aren't going to ruin your Relaxation Response. Just say to yourself, "Oh, well," and let the thoughts drift out of your mind. If they return, don't worry about them and don't try to fight them. Just keep repeating the word "one," breathing easily and rhythmically and keeping your muscles relaxed.

Continue for 10 to 20 minutes. When you finish, sit quietly for a while and then gradually open your eyes.

You'll feel like your "idle" has just been turned down to where it belongs. Just as with a car, you may not realize that your motor is racing until it's lowered. Then you can feel that the *energy* is still there, waiting to be called on, but there's less noise and shaking and smoke. You suddenly realize that what you had become habituated to accept as normal really wasn't, that the tension was abusing your body's most vital organs just as a racing auto motor damages the cylinders.

And if stress has you feeling not only tired, but anxious, helpless and a touch dissatisfied with life, the Relaxation Response may be of special value. Studies have shown that individuals who meditate regularly tend to become less anxious, more self-reliant and more self-fulfilled—traits that certainly boost our zest for life.

One of our editors first learned of this relaxation technique while reading Dr. Benson's book, *The Relaxation Response* (William Morrow, 1975). He tried a full session of meditation on a bus ride to New York. "The time was dusk, which is usually one of the most trying times of the day from the point of view of exhaustion, hunger and irritability," said our editor. "I was amazed at how mellow, relaxed and content I felt during and after that first meditation."

Use the Relaxation Response regularly to train yourself to relax, and you'll find that the moments that present great emotional challenges are much easier to handle. Even a minute or two of meditation at an especially overwrought moment can be a blessing. Once you get the hang of it, you can swing into a very relaxed state anytime you want to with just a few good breaths, almost like pushing a button.

In his book, Dr. Benson describes how some people work relaxation breaks into their lives. One businessman tells his secretary he's "in conference" late in the morning and takes no calls. When he travels, he uses the Relaxation Response in airplanes. A housewife takes a relaxation break in the morning after her husband has left for work and her children have gone to school. A college student arrives at the lecture hall 15 minutes early and practices the Response before class begins.

Relaxation Helps Cut Down on Coffee and Cigarettes

The Relaxation Response is of special value to people who use coffee and cigarettes to keep them going. Under the stress of a heavy academic schedule, and a fulltime job, one woman graduate student at Old Dominion University in Norfolk, Virginia, came to rely heavily on cigarettes and caffeine to keep herself alert. When her heartbeat consistently shot up to superhigh levels (tachycardia), her doctor told her the stimulants would have to go. Easier said than done, though. The woman had tried to cut down in the past, with no luck. After just three weeks of practicing Dr. Benson's Relaxation Response, however, she eventually cut down on coffee and quit smoking entirely—in spite of the added pressure of a final exam in the interim! And, as hoped, after one year her heartbeat had returned to normal (*Psychological Reports,* October, 1979).

So if you depend on either coffee (or tea) or cigarettes for regular pick-me-ups under stress, the Relaxation Response is worth a try. (For more on the anti-pep effects of coffee and cigarettes, see the chapter Why Coffee and Other Stimulants Don't Work.)

Deep Muscle Relaxation

This technique is similar to the Relaxation Response in a very general way, but is somewhat different in the specific manner in which it works. About 70 years ago, a young graduate student from Harvard had a profound insight: When we're under mental stress, we tense our muscles, and by tensing our muscles, we cause ourselves physical discomfort that tends to make our mental stress even worse. His name was Edmund Jacobson, and he went on to become a renowned psychiatrist who gradually perfected a technique for breaking this tense mind–tense muscle cycle. He called it Progressive Relaxation.

Psychologists and other health care professionals who've adopted or modified Jacobson's technique often call it deep muscle relaxation or, sometimes, full body relaxation. And it works by forcing us to focus in on how it actually *feels* to be physically relaxed.

As with the Relaxation Response, daily sessions of deep muscle relaxation lasting about 20 minutes are normally recommended, but once people get the hang of it, the sessions can be shortened and used in certain spur-of-the-moment situations—in a traffic jam or to cure pre-big-meeting jitters, for example. The technique has been enjoying something of a resurgence lately among psychologists and medical people.

The following version of deep muscle relaxation is taught at the Integral Health Services, a holistic medical center in Putnam, Connecticut.

1. Lie flat on your back, placing the feet about 18 inches apart. The hands should rest slightly away from the trunk, with the palms up.

2. Close your eyes and gently move all the different parts of the body to create a general feeling of relaxation.

3. Then start relaxing the body part by part. First concentrate on the right leg. Inhale and slowly raise the leg about one foot off the floor. Hold it fully tensed. After five seconds, exhale abruptly and

relax the muscles of the right leg, allowing it to fall to the floor on its own. Shake the leg gently from right to left, relax it fully, and forget about the existence of this leg.
4. Repeat this same process with the left leg, and then with both hands, one at a time.
5. Then bring the mind to the muscles of the pelvis, buttocks and anus. Tense them and relax. Once again, tense them and relax. Next, concentrate on your abdomen. Inhale deeply through the nose and bloat the abdomen. Hold your breath for five seconds and suddenly let the air burst out through the mouth, simultaneously relaxing all the muscles of the abdomen and diaphragm.
6. Move up to the chest region. Inhale deeply through the nose, bloating the chest. Hold your breath for five seconds and suddenly let the air out through the mouth while relaxing all the muscles of the chest and diaphragm.
7. Move on to the shoulders. Without moving the forearms off the floor, try to make the shoulders meet in front of the body. Then relax and let them drop to the floor.
8. Slowly, gently, turn the neck right and left, right and left, then back to center, mentally relaxing the neck muscles.
9. Coming to the facial muscles, move the jaw up and down, left and right a few times, then relax. Squeeze the lips together in a pout, then relax. Suck in the cheek muscles, then relax. Tense the tip of the nose, then relax. Wrinkle the forehead muscles, then relax.
10. Now you have relaxed all the muscles of the body. To make sure of this, allow your mind to wander over your entire body from the tips of the toes to the head, searching for any spots of tension. If you come across any spots of tension, concentrate upon this part and it will relax. If you do this mentally, without moving a muscle, you will notice that the part concerned obeys your command.

This is complete relaxation. Even your mind is at rest now. Be aware of your breath, which will keep flowing in and out quite freely and calmly. Observe your thoughts without trying to take your mind anywhere. You are a witness, not a body or a mind but an ocean of peace and tranquillity. Remain in this condition at least five minutes.

Do not become anxious about anything. When you decide to wake from this conscious sleep, do so quite slowly. Imagine that fresh energy is gently entering each part of your body, from the head down to the toes. Then slowly sit up. This exercise helps create a refreshed and peaceful feeling for the body and mind. Try to do this one to three times a day, especially upon arising and before retiring.

A modified version of this exercise can be performed sitting upright in a firm, comfortable chair. Seat yourself with your spine erect, your head upright and your jaw relaxed. Close your eyes and allow your entire body to relax and rest. Practice full deep breathing and hold this position for three to five minutes as you make a conscious effort to release all of the tension in your body and keep your mind still, focused and quiet. That variation is a perfect exercise to perform at work, in a bus, while sitting in the park or anywhere else when a relaxation break would be helpful.

Deep Breathing

Chances are you've never thought of breathing as a relaxation technique. But breathing—*deep* breathing—can unknot tension. *And* damp the fuse of anger. *And* smooth out a case of the jitters. In short, deep breathing can dissolve many of the physical effects of stress that can so easily weigh us down.

The most recent scientific evidence pointing to a link between breathing patterns and relaxation comes from the laboratory of Otto H. Schmitt, Ph.D., head of the biophysics laboratory at the University of Minnesota.

"It's possible that your heartbeat and breathing pattern together may show whether you are relaxed or tense," Dr. Schmitt told us. "Eventually, science may be able to confirm the idea that by changing your breathing patterns you can calm yourself or change your mental state," he said.

Dr. Schmitt didn't set out to investigate breathing. His aim was to produce perfect measurements of the heartbeat during diagnostic tests. But there was one problem. As the patient breathed during the test, the heartbeat changed. To tune out this "static," he connected patients to a minicomputer, which displayed their heartbeats and also instructed them when to inhale and when to exhale so an exact number of heartbeats would be included in each breath cycle.

"I succeeded in producing a standard heartbeat during the test," Dr. Schmitt told us, "but I also noticed that as a person followed the computer's instructions for breathing, he or she had a tendency to become more relaxed and calm, even to the point of falling asleep."

But you don't need a private computer to relax through breathing. Anyone can do this exercise at home, said Dr. Schmitt.

"Feel your pulse," he instructed. "Then inhale for two beats and exhale for three. If you inhale and exhale longer, you may even become more relaxed."

A refinement on the exercise is to actually feel your heartbeat without taking your pulse. "With practice, anyone can hear his heartbeat," said Dr. Schmitt.

"The relaxation that can be achieved by this breathing exercise reminded me of the claims of some yogis who say they can achieve a calm mental state through specific types of breathing. I thought, 'Perhaps my method of matching breathing and heartbeat is similar to the condition that yogis achieve through their breathing exercises.'"

Dr. Schmitt didn't have long to wait for an answer. News of his research traveled to Swami Rama, a yogi, founder of the Chicago-based Himalayan International Institute and author of a book on yogic breathing techniques.

In a meeting of East and West at Dr. Schmitt's laboratory, Swami Rama told the researcher that his patients were performing a type of "pranayam"—a yogic breathing exercise designed to calm the mind and relax the body.

What are the breathing exercises of pranayam? Well, there are all kinds. One exercise has you pinching one nostril shut while breathing through the other. In another, you push air in and out of your lungs forcefully and rapidly, using your diaphragm as a pump. But the simplest, most fundamental—and probably the best—yogic breathing exercise is deep breathing.

You can do deep breathing either sitting in a chair or lying down. The point is to have your back as straight as possible. But no straining. Your back should be straight, not rigid.

Now put your fingertips on your abdomen and notice how it moves when you normally inhale and exhale. It may not be moving at all! If you're tense or nervous, you may be breathing from your chest. But the healthiest, most natural breathing is when the abdomen slightly swells as you inhale and slightly contracts as you exhale. Babies breathe this way. And so do you—when you're as peaceful as a sleeping baby.

So the point in deep breathing is to do what comes naturally, but what the stress and strain of daily life may have inhibited.

Begin by breathing in slowly and evenly through your nostrils. In the first few sessions, keep your fingertips lightly on your abdomen and see how deep down into the abdomen you can breathe. Feel how your abdomen expands, then your rib cage, then your entire lungs.

To exhale, simply reverse the process, again breathing through your nostrils slowly and evenly. Finish the breath by gently contracting the abdomen and expelling the last of the stale air.

Don't strain. Never breathe beyond your capacity, trying to force air into your lungs. Just breathe rhythmically and easily. And try to take as long to exhale as you do to inhale. Do that by slowly counting to three as you inhale, and again to three as you exhale. As your breathing capacity improves, you can work slowly up to a higher count.

Try deep breathing the next time you're hit by the 5 P.M. blahs, or anytime you feel tired, tense and bored. Just take three or four deep breaths—and then take note of your livelier, calmer mood. Other great times for deep breathing are in the morning before you get out of bed and in the evening as you lie in bed before sleep. In the morning, it can give you a lift; in the evening, it can settle you gently into sleep.

How long should you deep breathe? For as long as is comfortable. But a minute or so of deep breathing should be the minimum for best results.

PART II

Supernutrition for Work and Play

Vitamins and Minerals That Combat Fatigue

CHAPTER 4

You may have an athletic friend or two who start out each day by downing a full complement of vitamin and mineral supplements. No doubt they have learned that the bodies of even highly trained athletes demand excellent nutrition to be able to run long distances or perform their best under the stress of exertion. Now, while most people are in a different league than hard-core athletes, the average office worker, laborer, student or family manager relies on some of the same nutrients to improve "performance." (After all, the laundry can seem like a decathlon to a pooped-out housekeeper.) So if everywhere you look you see work to be done—or pet projects you'd like to start or hobbies to pursue—but you can barely drag one foot after the other, don't tell yourself you're just not as young as you used to be. Instead, you'd probably be better off consulting a checklist of nutrients shown to relieve tiredness and boost productivity. And while any overall nutritional deficiency is likely to slow you down, certain nutrients are particularly important. Even a slight deficiency of any of those nutrients could be robbing you of vitality.

Potassium and Magnesium for Get-Up-and-Go

Potassium deficiency is a well-known hazard among long-distance runners and professional athletes. The mineral helps to cool muscles, and hours of exertion use it up. If it's not replaced, the result is chronic fatigue—even for a highly trained athlete. "When you lack potassium," says Gabe Mirkin, M.D., runner of

38

marathons and coauthor of *The Sportsmedicine Book* (Little, Brown, 1978), "you feel tired, weak and irritable."

But a potassium deficiency and the weakness that goes with it aren't limited to athletes. In one study, researchers randomly selected a group of people and measured their potassium intake. Those people with a deficient intake of potassium—60 percent of the men and 40 percent of the women in the study—had a weaker grip than those with a normal intake. And as potassium intake decreased, muscular strength decreased (*Journal of the American Medical Association*, October 6, 1979).

You could probably put up with a few days of that kind of weakness. But after a few months you feel terrible. "In chronic potassium deficit," writes a researcher who studied the mineral, "muscular weakness may persist for many months and be interpreted as being due to emotional disability" (*Minnesota Medicine*, June, 1965).

In other words, tiredness often means tired *muscles*— muscles that feel leaden or drained of energy. But it's not only a lack of potassium that hobbles muscles. A lack of magnesium, which helps muscles contract, can also cause tiredness.

But don't tell your doctor that. He's only been trained to recognize a *severe* deficiency of magnesium and the severe symptoms that go with it—a stumbling gait, depression and heart spasms. The typical M.D. would probably fail to spot a mild deficiency. It has only one noticeable symptom—chronic fatigue.

"A deficiency of magnesium is a common cause of fatigue," says Ray Wunderlich, M.D., a nutritionally oriented doctor from St. Petersburg, Florida.

But that fatigue can easily be cured. In one scientific study, 200 men and women who were tired during the day were given magnesium. In all but two cases, waking tiredness disappeared (*Second International Symposium on Magnesium*, June, 1976).

Sometimes, however, both potassium *and* magnesium levels dip too low, sapping our natural vitality. A doctor chose 100 of her chronically fatigued patients—84 women and 16 men, 1 in 5 of whom held a full or parttime job—and put them on a supplementary program of potassium and magnesium. Of the 100, 87 improved.

"The change was startling," writes Palma Formica, M.D., of Old Bridge, New Jersey. "They had become alert, cheerful, animated and energetic and walked with a lively step. They stated that sleep refreshed them as it had not done for months. Some said they could get along on 6 hours' sleep at night, whereas formerly they had not felt rested on 12 or more. Morning exhaustion had completely subsided.

"Almost all patients have undertaken new activities," she
notes. "Six who had not worked outside the home before obtained
parttime jobs. Two of the pregnant patients continued to work for
a time. Several of the husbands called and expressed appreciation

Table 1
FOOD SOURCES OF POTASSIUM

Food	Portion	Potassium (milligrams)
Potato	1 medium	782
Avocado	½	680
Raisins	½ cup	553
Sardines, drained solids	3 ounces	501
Flounder	3 ounces	498
Orange juice	1 cup	496
Squash, winter	½ cup	473
Tomato, raw	1	444
Banana	1	440
Milk, skim	1 cup	406
Salmon, fillet, fresh	3 ounces	378
Beans	½ cup	374
Buttermilk	1 cup	371
Milk, whole	1 cup	370
Cod	3 ounces	345
Sweet potato	1 medium	342
Beef liver	3 ounces	323
Apricots, dried	¼ cup	318
Turkey	3 ounces	312
Peach	1 medium	308
Apricots, fresh	3	301
Round steak, trimmed of fat	3 ounces	298
Haddock	3 ounces	297
Pork, trimmed of fat	3 ounces	283
Leg of lamb, trimmed of fat	3 ounces	274
Perch	3 ounces	243
Tuna, drained solids	3 ounces	225

SOURCES: Adapted from
Nutritive Value of American Foods in Common Units, Agriculture
Handbook No. 456, by Catherine F. Adams (Washington, D.C.: Agri-
cultural Research Service, U.S. Department of Agriculture, 1975).
Composition of Foods: Dairy and Egg Products, Agriculture Handbook
No. 8–1, by Consumer and Food Economics Institute (Washington, D.C.:
Agricultural Research Service, U.S. Department of Agriculture, 1976).

Table 2
FOOD SOURCES OF MAGNESIUM

Food	Portion	Magnesium (milligrams)
Soy flour	½ cup	155
Soybeans, dried	¼ cup	138
Buckwheat flour, light	½ cup	112
Black-eyed peas, dried	¼ cup	98
Almonds	¼ cup	96
Tofu (soybean curd)	3 ounces	95
Cashews	¼ cup	94
Lima beans, large, dried, raw	¼ cup	81
Brazil nuts	¼ cup	79
Pecans, halved	¼ cup	77
Kidney beans, dried	¼ cup	75
Whole wheat flour	½ cup	68
Shredded wheat	1 cup	67
Peanuts, roasted, chopped	¼ cup	63
Walnuts, black, chopped	¼ cup	60
Banana	1 medium	58
Beet greens, raw, chopped	1 cup	58
Avocado	½	56
Peanut butter	2 tablespoons	56
Peanut flour	¼ cup	54
Blackstrap molasses	1 tablespoon	52
Potato	1 medium	51
Oatmeal	1 cup	50
Spinach, raw, chopped	1 cup	48
Brown rice	¾ cup	42
Rye flour	½ cup	37
Swiss chard, raw, chopped	1 cup	36
Chestnuts	½ cup	33
Salmon, sockeye, drained solids	3 ounces	32
Collards, raw	1 cup	31
Milk, skim	1 cup	28
Wheat germ, raw	1 tablespoon	24
Ground beef, lean	3 ounces	21

SOURCES: Adapted from
Composition of Foods, Agriculture Handbook No. 8, rev. ed., by Bernice K. Watt and Annabel L. Merrill (Washington, D.C.: Agricultural Research Service, U.S. Department of Agriculture, 1975).
Composition of Foods: Dairy and Egg Products, Agriculture Handbook No. 8-1, by Consumer and Food Economics Institute (Washington, D.C.: Agricultural Research Service, U.S. Department of Agriculture, 1976).

of the physical improvement and consequent increase in emotional well-being of their wives" (*Current Therapeutic Research,* March, 1962).

Since many foods are rich in potassium (and since government regulations have put a lid on the amount of potassium allowed in nonprescription tablets), the best way to boost your intake of this mineral is through your diet. Apricots, bananas, beef, fish, milk, oranges, potatoes, raisins and tomatoes are some of the richest sources. Useful amounts of magnesium come from blackstrap molasses, brown rice, green leafy vegetables, nuts, peas, soybeans, whole wheat bread and other whole grain products. See tables 1 and 2 for more complete lists. If you feel you cannot meet your magnesium needs through diet alone, magnesium supplements in the form of magnesium gluconate and other compounds, plus dolomite (a combination of calcium and magnesium) are available.

Calcium Bolsters Stamina

Over the years, various research has shown that calcium has a strong influence on the power of muscles to contract. That being the case, it occurred to biologists at Old Dominion University in Norfolk, Virginia, that a calcium supplement added to the diet might very well increase stamina by prolonging muscle contraction. John H. Richardson, M.D., and two associates fed identical diets to 40 experimental rats for 60 days, but added 10 milligrams of calcium (equivalent to about 1,400 milligrams for people) to the drinking water of 20 of the rats. Half the animals in each group worked out on an exercise wheel for two weeks of the experimental period; the other half did not. At the conclusion of the experiment, the researchers measured muscle contractions in a lower leg muscle of all the rats with a special device called a myograph. "Both calcium and exercise were effective in prolonging time for the onset of fatigue in [this type of] muscle," reported Dr. Richardson and his co-workers. What's more, among the rats that exercised, muscles tired far less easily in those given calcium than in those not given calcium. "This study suggests that calcium given orally and exercise causes increased stamina as a result of [calcium's] effect in prolonging time for the onset of muscle fatigue," the biologists concluded (*Journal of Sports Medicine,* June, 1980).

Dairy products are good sources of calcium, but not the only sources. (See table 3.) As for supplements, bone meal provides generous amounts of calcium, and dolomite supplies both calcium and magnesium. Calcium supplements such as calcium

Table 3
FOOD SOURCES OF CALCIUM

Food	Portion	Calcium (milligrams)
Swiss cheese	2 ounces	544
Yogurt, skim-milk	1 cup	452
Provolone cheese	2 ounces	428
Monterey Jack cheese	2 ounces	424
Cheddar cheese	2 ounces	408
Muenster cheese	2 ounces	406
Colby cheese	2 ounces	388
Brick cheese	2 ounces	382
Sardines, Atlantic, drained solids	3 ounces	371
Mozzarella cheese	2 ounces	366
American cheese	2 ounces	348
Milk, skim	1 cup	302
Buttermilk	1 cup	285
Limburger cheese	2 ounces	282
Salmon, sockeye, drained solids	3 ounces	274
Dandelion greens, cooked	½ cup	147
Pizza, cheese	⅛ of 14-inch pie	144
Blackstrap molasses	1 tablespoon	137
Soy flour	½ cup	132
Collards, cooked	½ cup	110
Tofu (soybean curd)	3 ounces	109
Kale, cooked	½ cup	103
Mustard greens, cooked	½ cup	97
Watercress, finely chopped	½ cup	95
Almonds	¼ cup	83
Chick-peas, dried	¼ cup	75
Parmesan cheese	1 tablespoon	69
Broccoli, cooked	½ cup	68
Soybeans	½ cup	66
Artichoke	1 medium bud	61
Filberts	¼ cup	60
Eggs	2 large	56
Cottage cheese, dry-curd, uncreamed	½ cup	23

SOURCES: Adapted from
Nutritive Value of American Foods in Common Units, Agriculture Handbook No. 456, by Catherine F. Adams (Washington, D.C.: Agricultural Research Service, U.S. Department of Agriculture, 1975).

(continued)

Table 3—continued
Composition of Foods: Dairy and Egg Products, Agriculture Handbook
No. 8-1, by Consumer and Food Economics Institute (Washington, D.C.:
Agricultural Research Service, U.S. Department of Agriculture, 1976).

gluconate, calcium carbonate, calcium lactate and calcium phos-
phate are also available. And if your drinking water is hard, that
means you get a little calcium and magnesium along with it.

Iron Boosts Work Capacity

Not all cases of chronic fatigue are caused by a lack of
potassium, magnesium or calcium. In fact, a good many are
caused by a lack of iron.

Iron helps form hemoglobin, the substance in red blood cells
that carries oxygen from your lungs to the rest of your body. If
there's not enough hemoglobin and that oxygen supply is reduced,
you have apathy, tiredness and irritability—the symptoms of iron
deficiency anemia. But you don't need to have out-and-out
anemia to suffer fatigue from a lack of iron.

"A deficiency of iron may be present when blood hemoglobin levels fall within normal limits," Dr. Wunderlich explained.
"This syndrome of iron deficiency without anemia," he
continued, "is an exceedingly important cause of fatigue."

Iron deficiency creeps up on you. Menstrual periods drain
iron. Pregnancies sap it. Reducing diets cut down your intake.
Before you know it, every cell of your body is dragging.

One study shows just how slow you go compared to someone who's not iron deficient. Researchers studied the "physical
work capacity" of 75 women, some anemic, some not. The
anemic women could stay on a treadmill an average of eight
minutes less than the nonanemic group. None of the anemic
women could perform under "highest work load" conditions,
while all of the nonanemic group could. During a work test, the
heartbeat of those with anemia rose to an average of 176 per
minute; for nonanemics, heartbeat rose to just 130. Levels of
lactate, a chemical in the muscles that is linked to fatigue, were
almost twice as high in the anemic group (*American Journal of
Clinical Nutrition,* June, 1977).

But relief from iron deficiency–induced fatigue is simple.
Replace the iron.

Workers on an Indonesian rubber plantation were paid by
productivity, and researchers found that those who were anemic

earned the least. But after two months of iron supplementation, the previously anemic workers had normal levels of iron and earned the same amount as those free from anemia (*American Journal of Clinical Nutrition,* April, 1979).

What's more, extra iron may improve work performance even in the absence of anemia, according to researcher Per

Table 4
FOOD SOURCES OF IRON

Food	Portion	Iron (milligrams)
Beef liver	3 ounces	7.5
Blackstrap molasses	1 tablespoon	3.2
Roast beef	3 ounces	3.1
Ground beef, lean	3 ounces	3.0
Lima beans, dried, cooked	½ cup	2.9
Sunflower seeds	¼ cup	2.6
Soybeans	½ cup	2.5
Prunes	½ cup	2.2
Turkey, dark meat	3 ounces	2.0
Apricots, dried	¼ cup	1.8
Broccoli, raw	1 stalk	1.7
Spinach, raw, chopped	1 cup	1.7
Almonds, slivered	¼ cup	1.6
Peas, fresh, cooked	½ cup	1.5
Beet greens, cooked	½ cup	1.4
Brewer's yeast	1 tablespoon	1.4
Raisins	¼ cup	1.3
Kidney beans, dried	¼ cup	1.1
Turkey, light meat	3 ounces	1.1
Chicken, white meat	3 ounces	1.0
Endive or escarole, shredded	1 cup	1.0
Cod	3 ounces	0.9
Haddock	3 ounces	0.9

SOURCES: Adapted from
Nutritive Value of American Foods in Common Units, Agricultural Handbook No. 456, by Catherine F. Adams (Washington, D.C.: Agricultural Research Service, U.S. Department of Agriculture, 1975).
Composition of Foods: Poultry Products, Agriculture Handbook No. 8–5, by Consumer and Food Economics Institute (Washington, D.C.: Science and Education Administration, U.S. Department of Agriculture, 1979).

Ericsson at the departments of medicine and clinical physiology, University Hospital, Uppsala, Sweden. A group of healthy people aged 58 to 71 took 120 milligrams of iron a day for three months. Work capacity—measured by how long they could ride on a bicyclelike machine—went up by 4 percent in the men and by 12 percent in the women (*Acta Medica Scandinavica*, vol. 188, 1970).

A bachelor who overcame fatigue by taking iron (and potassium) wrote to tell *Prevention* magazine:

> Over the past couple of years, I've been a victim of chronic fatigue. This is due in part to my job. Currently I work for the Philadelphia Inquirer as a driver-delivery man. Between my hours (8 P.M. to 5 A.M.) and the nature of the job, I've found getting proper rest sometimes impossible. In addition to my job, I'm very active athletically. It's not unusual for me to jog four or five times a week, from two to six miles at a time. On top of all that, I'm responsible for keeping my apartment, cooking and doing laundry.
>
> To help combat some of my eating deficiencies, I'd been taking selected vitamins and minerals. However, potassium and iron were not among them. Well, since adding those two to my daily intake, I've felt totally rejuvenated. I feel physically stronger and mentally clearer. I'm sleeping sounder and feeling refreshed when awakening. In the past I could be in bed nine or ten hours and still arise tired.

See Table 4 for a list of iron-rich foods. Iron supplements, in the form of ferrous sulfate or ferrous gluconate, are also available. We'd like to mention, too, that eating meat or some form of vitamin C (in food or supplement form) can triple your absorption of iron and help you benefit from that mineral.

Vitamins Prevent Slowdowns

While low iron is often the main cause of "tired blood," iron is only one of the nutrients that help produce a steady stream of new blood cells from our bone marrow—new cells that keep us feeling fit as a fiddle.

Folate

Without the B complex vitamin called folate, the body cannot manufacture some of the molecular building blocks of DNA. The DNA molecule, in turn, is the key to cell division. So less folate means less DNA, which means a slowdown in the creation of new cells—including oxygen-carrying red blood cells. Folate deficiency can easily lead to a type of anemia called megaloblastic anemia, in which the body produces abnormally large and poorly formed red blood cells.

Folate deficiency itself can trigger a wide range of symptoms. Sleeplessness, irritability, forgetfulness and depression are associated with acute deficiency. When the deficiency gives rise to megaloblastic anemia, lethargy, weakness and loss of color result.

Like iron, folate is a nutrient many people don't get enough of in their food. "Evidence is accumulating that folacin [folate] deficiency may be more widespread than previously suspected." That was the conclusion of a team of University of Florida and University of Miami researchers who recently studied blood samples from 193 elderly, low-income volunteers in the Coconut Grove section of Miami, Florida. Knowing that they would discover a high rate of nutrition-related anemia (an abnormally low concentration of red blood cells or hemoglobin) in this group, the researchers hoped to single out the *cause* of the anemia. Surprisingly, the missing link wasn't iron. It was folate.

Based on the folate content of their red blood cells, 60 percent of the volunteers fell into the category of "high risk" for folate deficiency, and another 11 percent evidenced a "medium risk." Fourteen percent were frankly anemic. At the same time, "the iron status of these elderly people was normal and indicates that the anemia was not due to a dietary iron deficiency.

"These findings . . . point out the fallacy of the rather widespread assumption that anemia always reflects dietary iron deficiency," the Florida study noted. "It is important to reassess the true incidence of iron deficiency worldwide in view of mounting evidence of the extent of folacin deficiency" (*American Journal of Clinical Nutrition,* November, 1979).

A glance at the diets of the elderly volunteers revealed an absence of foods rich in folate. Only 17 percent of the group said they ate fresh vegetables, and—in spite of the abundance of fresh oranges and grapefruit in Florida—only 30 percent reported eating citrus fruits. Some of these people also customarily boiled their vegetables for several hours, thereby destroying most of the folate.

Beef liver is a good source of folate. It's also a primary source of other nutrients that the blood thrives on, such as vitamin B_{12}, iron, riboflavin and vitamin A. Folate can also be found in brewer's yeast, legumes of various kinds and most other vegetables. (See table 5.) Whole grain bread, meat and eggs are moderately good sources of folate.

Table 5
FOOD SOURCES OF FOLATE

Food	Portion	Folate (micrograms)
Brewer's yeast	1 tablespoon	313
Orange juice	1 cup	136
Beef liver	3 ounces	123
Black-eyed peas	½ cup	100
Romaine lettuce	1 cup	98
Beets	½ cup	67
Broccoli	½ cup	50
Cantaloupe	¼ melon	41
Brussels sprouts	4	28

SOURCE: Adapted from
"Folacin in Selected Foods," by Betty P. Perloff and R. R. Butrum, *Journal of the American Dietetic Association,* vol. 70, February, 1977.

The elderly, with their tea-and-toast diets, aren't the only ones who risk folate deficiency. Teenagers, with their cola-and-fries diets, need extra folate to keep up with their accelerated growth rate. But many of them aren't getting it.

In a study of 199 12- to 16-year-olds in the Liberty City section of Miami, the same group of Florida researchers found approximately *50 percent* of these low-income adolescents to be deficient in folate and about 10 percent deficient in iron.

Again, in a paper presented in April, 1980, to the Federation of American Societies for Experimental Biology, the researchers stressed that the importance of folate shouldn't be eclipsed by an overemphasis on iron. "The incidence of folic acid [folate] deficiency during adolescence has not been widely studied," they said. "In fact, the potential for a folic acid deficiency is often ignored. If anemia is present, it is generally assumed to be due to an iron deficiency."

Researcher James Dinning, Ph.D., calls folate deficiency among teenagers a "high-priority area," and believes that it may affect more people than, for example, high cholesterol. "Folate deficiency could be the major problem in this country," Dr. Dinning said.

Of particular concern was the impact of low folate levels on adolescent girls, especially in light of the high rate of teenage pregnancies in the United States. "A long-term folic acid deficiency prior to pregnancy has been found . . . to adversely affect the outcome of pregnancy," warned Dr. Dinning.

Besides anemia, folate deficiency has recently been linked to neurological problems. Researchers at the laboratory of neuroanatomy at McGill University in Montreal, Canada, found that folate supplementation relieved mild depression, fatigue and abnormal intellectual or nerve function in certain people. These symptoms appeared even *before* the folate deficiency was severe enough to show up on a routine blood test (*Nature,* March, 1979).

Serge Gauthier, M.D., one of the McGill researchers, told us that the neurological problems stemming from lack of folate are mild, "but since it's a common deficiency, it's worth looking into." His research group suggested that shortages of vitamins such as folate can influence behavior by decreasing the synthesis of neurotransmitters, the molecules that relay brain messages. Dr. Gauthier warned that older people are particularly vulnerable to the neurological effects of folate deficiency.

Vitamin B12

You can't talk about folate without mentioning vitamin B_{12}. Without B_{12}, the folate needed for DNA synthesis remains trapped in a form the body can't use. Vitamin B_{12}, however, is more than folate's understudy. It plays an important role on its own. It can relieve tiredness. Twenty-eight men and women who complained of tiredness but who had no physical problems were given B_{12} and then asked to evaluate its effect. For many of the 28, the vitamin not only made them feel less fatigued, but also improved their appetite, sleep and general well-being (*British Journal of Nutrition,* September, 1973).

B_{12} is an unusual vitamin in that it's not found in *any* vegetables, fruits, grains or grain products. But meat, poultry, fish and eggs all supply plenty of the vitamin. (See table 6.)

Pantothenate

Still another B complex vitamin helps us tire less easily—because it helps us stand up under stress.

Way back in the 30s, researchers had already discovered that rats fed a pantothenate-deficient diet reacted poorly to stress while rats given extra pantothenate coped with stress better.

In one study, rats were divided into three groups. One group got a diet deficient in pantothenate. Another group got a diet adequate in pantothenate. The third group got a diet high in this vitamin. Then all the rats were put in cold water and made to swim until they were exhausted. The pantothenate-deficient rats

Table 6
FOOD SOURCES OF VITAMIN B₁₂

Food	Portion	Vitamin B₁₂ (micrograms)
Beef liver	3 ounces	93.5
Lamb	3 ounces	2.6
Beef	3 ounces	2.0
Tuna, drained	3 ounces	1.8
Yogurt	1 cup	1.5
Haddock	3 ounces	1.4
Swiss cheese	2 ounces	1.0
Milk, whole	1 cup	0.9
Cottage cheese	½ cup	0.7
Egg	1	0.7
Cheddar cheese	2 ounces	0.4
Chicken, light meat	3 ounces	0.4

SOURCES: Adapted from
Pantothenic Acid, Vitamin B₆ and Vitamin B₁₂ in Foods, Home Economics Research Report No. 36, by Martha Louise Orr (Washinton, D.C.: Agricultural Research Service, U.S. Department of Agriculture, 1969).
Composition of Foods: Dairy and Egg Products, Agriculture Handbook No. 8–1, by Consumer and Food Economics Institute (Washington, D.C.: Agricultural Research Service, U.S. Department of Agriculture, 1976).

swam an average of 16 minutes. The "adequate" group did better: they swam an average of 29 minutes. But the rats with a diet high in pantothenate swam an average of 62 minutes.

And pantothenate can keep *people* in the swim, too. In 1952, Elaine Ralli and her co-worker, Mary Dumm, researchers in the department of medicine at the New York University–Bellevue Medical Center in New York City, tested the antistress effects of pantothenate on humans. The researchers immersed a group of normal men in 48°F water for eight minutes. Precise chemical measurements of the men's blood and urine were taken before and at intervals after the stress. Then, for six weeks, the men received 10 grams of calcium pantothenate (a common form of pantothenate) every day. At the end of six weeks they were again immersed and the same measurements were taken.

Usually, stress causes a decrease in some of the white blood cells that protect the body against infection. After taking the pantothenate, the men had a "less pronounced" drop in these white blood cells. Also, levels of ascorbic acid (vitamin C)—a nutrient burned up by stress—were "significantly higher." And the men excreted less uric acid, a sign that the body had not undergone as much wear and tear. Importantly, they also had lower cholesterol levels (*Vitamins and Hormones,* vol. 11, 1953).

PANTOTHENATE HELPS YOU BOUNCE BACK AFTER SURGERY.
One stressful cause of fatigue is surgery. Pantothenate is one of the nutrients (including zinc and vitamins A and C, most notably) that help us sail through the postoperative days.

Fifty patients undergoing abdominal surgery were given 500 milligrams of panthenol—a substance similar to pantothenate—on the day of surgery and for five days afterward. Another 50 patients were not given panthenol.

The group receiving panthenol had quicker recoveries, with less nausea and vomiting—"a more benign postoperative course," in the words of the researchers conducting the study (*American Journal of Surgery,* January, 1959).

Pantothenate is found in almost all foods. But Mother Nature's pantry—brimming with vegetables, lean meats, whole grains, fruits, nuts and seeds—is a far cry from the pantry in most modern households where canned, frozen and highly processed foods crowd out the real thing.

In other words, much pantothenate is lost during canning and other forms of refining and processing. When fresh vegetables are frozen, pantothenate gets the cold shoulder—the vegetables lose anywhere from 37 to 57 percent of this vitamin. Canned vegetables lose from 46 to 78 percent of their pantothenate. Processed and refined grains—the kind used in baking most of the breads, cakes, cookies, crackers and chips sold in supermarkets—lose 37 to 74 percent of this nutrient. Processed meats do no better, losing 50 to 75 percent (*American Journal of Clinical Nutrition,* May, 1971).

So your best ammunition in the war against stress-caused fatigue is unrefined pantothenate-rich foods—like brown rice, whole wheat products, oats, brewer's yeast and eggs.

Eating for Daylong Energy

Someone once said, "Eat breakfast like a king, lunch like a prince, and supper like a pauper." Whether that person knew it or not, that's the kind of meal pattern that can help maintain daylong energy. Yet many of us do exactly the opposite: with most of the day's work in front of us, we have little more than coffee and a roll at breakfast (if that), grab a hurried lunch, and too often end the day with a heavy meal. But if we spread those three meals out into six—or even eight—we would eat more of our daily calories earlier, and the many feedings would help buoy us up throughout the day.

Gorging Is Out, Nibbling Is In

New studies are proving that nibbling—eating multiple small meals—is far more healthful than gorging. In a study conducted by Charlotte M. Young, Ph.D., and co-workers at Cornell University, 11 obese young men were placed on a 1,800-calorie diet. The calories were provided in either one, three or six meals each day. Cholesterol levels were significantly higher in participants eating only one meal a day. Cholesterol levels dropped at three meals a day and were reduced further with six meals a day. Participants eating only one meal a day also had significantly higher levels of fats in the blood and their glucose tolerance (ability to metabolize sugar) was lower (*Journal of the American Dietetic Association,* November, 1971).

A similar experiment conducted at the University of Wisconsin, Madison, also showed the physiological benefit of

nibbling over gorging. Participants ate two meals a day for four weeks. The first meal was at 8 A.M. and consisted of one-eighth of their total food intake for the day. The second meal was at 5 P.M. and consisted of the remaining seven-eighths of their total daily intake. When the participants were fed sugar, they exhibited abnormally high insulin responses. (Insulin is the hormone that keeps blood sugar levels normal.)

The participants were then given eight meals a day in equal portions between the hours of 8 A.M. and 10 P.M. On the nibbling program, their insulin responses to sugar returned to normal within one week. After four weeks, their insulin values were even *lower* than when they began the experiment, a sign that their blood sugar metabolism was very efficient (*American Journal of Clinical Nutrition*, August, 1973).

Nibbling for Pep

Those two studies also show that one of the biggest bonuses of eating smaller meals may be the positive effect on our energy levels. In both studies, eating one very large meal a day (as opposed to several smaller ones) seemed to produce either glucose intolerance or abnormal insulin responses. And fatigue— especially the kind where your energy levels seem to yo-yo throughout the day—has been associated with such blood sugar problems. So it's possible that eating several small meals a day may help to smooth out some of the ups and downs in blood sugar and energy levels that can accompany widely spaced, large meals.

"Fatigue is a very subjective thing," said Dorothy J. Pringle, Ph.D., professor of nutritional science, who helped conduct the second nibbling experiment. "We couldn't measure fatigue in our subjects. But after they ate the evening meal consisting of seven-eights of the day's calories, the participants complained of sleepiness. They went home and slept an hour or two. At other times, we heard no such complaints from them.

"Now, no one has studied the specific effects of meal patterns on fatigue and blood sugar, so I can't say whether or not their tiredness was related to blood sugar. But on the other hand, ask most people on the street and they'll say they feel better after they've had a bite to eat—or they feel groggy after eating a large meal."

That opinion is seconded by Milton Fried, M.D., director of the Fried Medical Clinic in Atlanta, Georgia.

We asked Dr. Fried if he had any general advice for the great sleepy public. "I would advise anyone who wanted to stay alert after eating simply never to overeat at any one meal," he said. "You just can't think clearly and digest a big meal at the same time because the digestive organs shift blood away from the brain."

DRIVERS TAKING A BREAK
SHOULD TAKE A BITE

When you're taking a break during that interminable car trip to the beach this summer, the pause that refreshes best should include a hearty snack. So claim Swedish psychologists who recently tested the effects of food breaks vs. rest breaks on motoring ability when driving long distances. The researchers found that no matter how long the pit stop, only fueling up with a meal seemed to improve driving performances. And there seemed to be no difference in driving performance between a rest break of 15 minutes or an hour (*Journal of Applied Psychology*, March 24, 1980).

Speaking of digestion, recent experiments conducted by David L. Trout, Ph.D., of the U.S. Department of Agriculture's Nutrition Institute in Beltsville, Maryland, suggest that nibblers also have a slower gastric (stomach) emptying rate (GER) than gorgers—and a slower GER may mean less overeating. Dr. Trout fed one group of rats one large meal a day while the other group was fed the equivalent in four smaller but equal meals at six-hour intervals. The single-meal group had a higher GER than the others. When the large meal was reduced slightly, the GER was lowered but was *still* higher than that in rats eating four regular meals each day.

"When released by the stomach into the intestine, carbohydrates and fat are rapidly absorbed," Dr. Trout told us. "How rapidly that absorption takes place is dependent upon how rapidly the materials are made available by the stomach. If the gastric emptying rate is too fast, the carbohydrates are synthesized to fat at a faster degree, and the subject is ready for more food too early." According to these findings, nibblers may be less likely to feel pangs of hunger.

Dr. Trout expresses concern about American dietary habits which tend to avoid breakfast, limit lunch and emphasize dinner. "The effects on a person's insulin status with those eating patterns would worry me very much," he said. "I believe that several small meals a day are preferable. The primary concern is that *no* meal should be particularly large."

To stretch three square meals into six smaller meals, have breakfast, lunch and dinner as you customarily do. Then set, say 10:00–10:30 A.M., 3:00–3:30 P.M. and 9:00 P.M. or so as your "pick-me-up" breaks. As for *what* to eat, please read on.

Subtract Sugar, Add Protein

As it turns out, *what* we eat is just as important to energy levels as *how much* and *when*.

Take breakfast, for instance. Samuel J. Arnold, M.D., from Morristown, New Jersey, surveyed his patients who complained of fatigue and fluid retention, and found that 88 percent of the women and 67 percent of the men ate a poor breakfast or no breakfast at all. But those combined symptoms did not plague anyone who usually ate a high-protein breakfast. Dr. Arnold advised his tired patients to eat high-protein breakfasts, including eggs, fish, meat, cheese or brewer's yeast, and to reduce their intake of sugar, bread and cereal. All of the men and 95 percent of the women who persisted in their high-protein breakfasting reported substantial improvement. In some instances, the reduction in symptoms was "dramatic" (*Medical Tribune,* April 21, 1976).

While hearty breakfasts may have been popular with our grandparents, today's breakfasts are often devoured on the way out the door. The first meal of the day may be a chocolate-coated breakfast bar claiming to be nutritionally equivalent to a poached egg on toast, bacon and a glass of tomato juice. That same breakfast bar is less likely to advertise the fact that it is anywhere from 44 to 70 percent carbohydrate. Most of that carbohydrate is sugar in the form of sucrose, sorbitol, dextrose, lactose, glycerin and refiner's syrup.

And contrary to popular propaganda, sugar is *not* a "quick energy food." True, sugar (and all carbohydates) break down into glucose, the blood sugar that fuels the body. But the trick is to keep your body's engine running on all its cylinders by having enough glucose. The way to do that is definitely *not* by eating sugar, however.

Why not, if that's what the body runs on?

The answer is that the body is designed to run on a more or less steady, balanced supply of blood sugar. And to keep that supply smooth, the body has a regulating system—just like most cars have carburetors to control the burning of gasoline. What would happen to your car if you just dumped a gallon of fuel into the cylinders? It would be flooded. The same sort of thing happens in the body when you eat too much sugar. Within minutes after that sugar-coated cereal or that Continental breakfast of pastry leaves the plate, most of it breaks down into glucose and floods the bloodstream. The body's glucose-regulating system (the pancreas) gets the alarm and tries to lower the glucose level by releasing extra amounts of insulin, a hormone that causes glucose to be withdrawn from the blood and stored. But the high-sugar, high-refined-carbohydrate meal continues to overstimulate the pancreas until, not too long after the initial "sugar kick," the blood sugar drops to the point where the body literally runs out of fuel to burn.

To avoid overstimulating the pancreas, it is necessary to avoid sugar and refined carbohydrates. Replace them with protein-rich foods like fish, meat, milk, eggs and cheese. Protein (half of it, anyway) is digested into energy-producing glucose—but more slowly than carbohydrates. So the glucose will enter your blood a little at a time over a longer period—until your next snack or meal, if you eat enough protein.

There's still another reason why protein is part of a good food formula for open-eyed alertness. Protein is made up of various combinations of amino acids. "All the amino acids are competing with each other for entry into the brain," explains associate professor of pharmacology Miodrag Radulovacki, M.D., Ph.D., from his lab at the University of Illinois College of Medicine. In the case of drowsiness and wakefulness, says Dr. Radulovacki, we are concerned with the amino acids tryptophan and tyrosine. If tryptophan gets to the brain first, a group of neurotransmitters called catecholamines decrease, promoting drowsiness. If the other of the two amino acids, tyrosine, reaches the brain, though, catecholamines increase, promoting wakefulness.

So how do we help get tyrosine to our brains? By emphasizing protein-rich foods over carbohydrates. In one of a series of experiments, Richard J. Wurtman, M.D., and John D. Fernstrom, Ph.D., fed laboratory animals a single meal composed of 40 percent protein. The result? Tyrosine went up and so did catecholamines. "These observations," say Drs. Wurtman and Fernstrom, "suggest that . . . catecholamine-containing brain neurons are normally under specific dietary control" (*American Journal of Clinical Nutrition*, June, 1975).

Meat, fish, eggs, milk and cheese are our most concentrated sources of protein, but plant foods can also supply useful amounts. (See table 7.) Most adult women need about 44 grams of protein a day and most adult men, 56 grams.

Table 7
SOME SOURCES OF PROTEIN

Food	Portion	Protein (grams)
Chicken, light meat	3 ounces	28
Flounder	3 ounces	26
Cod	3 ounces	25
Chicken, dark meat	3 ounces	25
Ham, lean, trimmed of fat	3 ounces	25
Turkey, light meat	3 ounces	25
Prime rib of beef, trimmed of fat	3 ounces	24
Tuna, drained solids	3 ounces	24
Turkey, dark meat	3 ounces	24
Ground beef, lean	3 ounces	23
Ground beef, regular	3 ounces	23
Salmon, sockeye	3 ounces	23
Beef liver	3 ounces	22
Halibut	3 ounces	22
Sardines	3 ounces	20
Mackerel	3 ounces	19
Scallops	3 ounces	18
Haddock	3 ounces	17
Yogurt, skim-milk	1 cup	14
Cottage cheese, dry-curd	½ cup	12
Soybeans	½ cup	10
Yogurt, whole-milk	1 cup	9
Lentils	½ cup	8
Buttermilk	1 cup	8
Milk, skim	1 cup	8
Milk, whole	1 cup	8
Navy (pea) beans	½ cup	8
Split peas	½ cup	8
Kidney beans	½ cup	7
Tofu (soybean curd)	3 ounces	7
Lima beans	½ cup	6
Egg, hard-cooked	1	6
Brewer's yeast	1 tablespoon	3

SOURCES: Adapted from
Nutritive Value of American Foods in Common Units, Agriculture Handbook No. 456, by Catherine F. Adams (Washington, D.C.: Agricultural Research Service, U.S. Department of Agriculture, 1975).

(continued)

Table 7—continued
Composition of Foods: Poultry Products, Handbook No. 8-5, by Consumer and Food Economics Institute (Washington, D.C.: Science and Education Administration, U.S. Department of Agriculture, 1979).
Composition of Foods: Dairy and Egg Products, Handbook No. 8-1, by Consumer and Food Economics Institute (Washington, D.C.: Agricultural Research Service, U.S. Department of Agriculture, 1976).

The Art of Healthful Snacking

As long as you continue to eat the same number of calories a day as you customarily do, you won't gain weight eating from

POPCORN—THE PERFECT SNACK

For a snack, what could be better than popcorn?

Popcorn gives you energy without loading you full of sugar. It also contains fiber, which helps regulate blood sugar levels.

And a handful has only 6 calories. Compare that to the 114 calories in only 10 potato chips, and the 257 in a bowl of ice cream. Even 10 measly jelly beans have 104 calories.

Popcorn is best fresh, and it's simple to make. In a medium-size pot, heat one tablespoon of oil. (One popcorn lover we know uses different oils for a change of taste. Try peanut, corn or safflower oil.) Cover the bottom of the pot with a single layer of popcorn kernels—but not too much, because just a small amount will fill the pot. Then cover with a lid. Move the pot constantly to avoiding burning the corn. When the corn starts popping—in about a minute—turn the heat down slightly and continue shaking the pot over the heat until the kernels stop popping. Remove from heat.

You're now on your way to having a dynamite, wholesome snack.

But before you get to putting melted butter all over your treat, you might want to try some less fattening toppings.

Herbs and spices add *no* calories and they taste great. Try adding one or a combination of the following: garlic powder, chili powder, chives, basil, curry powder, cinnamon, dill—or Parmesan cheese if you can afford the extra calories.

Popcorn isn't just for the movies, either.

Pop a batch of corn, brown-bag it, and take it to work with you for midmorning energy-restoring munchies. Or stash some under the dash when you start out on your next all-day auto trip.

time to time during the day. "A person is not going to get any more or less fat by eating just one large meal or fewer smaller ones," said Gilbert A. Leveille, Ph.D., chairman of the department of food science and human nutrition at Michigan State University in East Lansing. "Whether a person eats one large meal or the equivalent in 16 small meals, the calories are used by the body with the same degree of efficiency."

Dr. Leveille has been researching meal patterns since the early 1960s. In a recent experiment, he divided rats into two groups. The first group was allowed to eat their food for only two hours a day. The second group was given the exact same amount of food, but a special feeding device provided it in smaller portions, which they nibbled throughout the day. "At the end of the experiment, there was absolutely no difference in weight between the two groups," said Dr. Leveille. When they are given precisely the same amount of food, nibblers and gorgers will come out even. The nibblers won't be fatter at all.

So it doesn't seem to matter how often we eat, but *what* we eat that determines what we weigh. Gorgers who may want to reform and enjoy the benefits of nibbling at smaller meals should remember a very important rule: eating more frequently does not mean snacking on junk.

Herbivorous (non-meat-eating) animals in natural settings nibble all day on fibrous vegetation, fruits or starchy roots. But with all of our artificially enriched and presweetened food products, humans tend to associate nibbling with high-calorie, low-bulk foods like candy bars, cakes, cookies and sweetened beverages. In order to benefit fully from multiple meals, we must include high-bulk, low-calorie foods like raw vegetables and fresh fruits along with the high-protein foods listed earlier. Here are a few suggestions to get you started on junk-free snacking for daylong energy:

■ Eat half your sandwich at midmorning, the rest with lunch.

■ Save half your meat from dinner (chicken, turkey, meatloaf and so on) for a late-night snack.

■ Have one scrambled egg instead of two at breakfast, and allow yourself a hard-boiled egg at midmorning or midafternoon. Or make up a batch of tangy pickled eggs to keep in the fridge for a quick dose of protein.

■ Blend fruit and yogurt for a late-afternoon "fruit shake." A refreshing breakfast drink, too!

■ Cut up cantaloupe, peaches, strawberries or oranges and top with a dollop of plain yogurt. Sprinkle on some chopped Brazil nuts, wheat germ or raisins.

■ Lightly toast whole wheat pita bread and spread with chopped liver. Or spread with ricotta cheese and top with a slice of tomato sprinkled with basil.

■ Spread chopped liver on celery stalks.

■ Combine carbonated water with fruit concentrate (mixed to taste) for a "fruit soda."

■ Try skewered chunks of banana rolled in wheat germ.

■ Make a "coffee table mix" of raisins, sunflower seeds and chopped walnuts.

Other handy, wholesome snacks are:

Apple slices or celery stalks with peanut butter
Bran or fruit muffins
Crackers with sesame butter (tahini) or Swiss cheese
Sunflower or pumpkin seeds
Tomato juice and other vegetable juices
Unsalted nuts (if you can afford the calories).

Why Coffee and Other Stimulants Don't Work

CHAPTER **6**

- An estimated 16 million Americans drink six or more cups of coffee a day.
- Nearly 40 percent of adult men smoke, and the number of women smokers is on the rise.
- Fifty-five percent of us are regular drinkers of alcohol—and 89 percent of a group of Fortune 500 executives surveyed recently qualified as moderate to heavy imbibers.

Would you drink as much coffee as you do if you thought it was slowing you down? Would you smoke cigarettes if you thought they were impairing your powers of concentration? Would you drink as much alcohol if you knew that every high is actually a low, slowing down some part of your body?

If you're going to use stimulants, keep one basic concept in mind: what goes up must come down.

"The person who has come to rely on pharmacological crutches has created a seesaw existence which finds him on top of a mountain or down in a valley. And fatigue . . . is his constant companion," according to M. F. Graham, M.D. (*Inner Energy,* Sterling, 1979).

Why fatigue?

Because stimulants (and we're going to include alcohol in this classification for its ability to loosen inhibitions) give us energy without giving us adequate fuel. Stimulants increase nearly all vital body functions—including producing a rapid rise in blood sugar—but that's *all* they do. They give us no sustenance. And worse yet, they give us no reliable feedback on when we should rest. In other words, we're using stimulants to give us **61** energy that isn't there—and draining ourselves in the process. No wonder we're pooped.

The Ups and Downs of Caffeine

Caffeine is a good example. The amount of caffeine in one or two cups of instant coffee (from 50 to 200 milligrams) is enough to:

- stimulate all parts of the brain,
- widen coronary arteries and pulmonary vessels,
- increase heart rate and force of contraction,
- increase the secretion of stomach acids,
- step up kidney (and hence bladder) action,
- increase overall metabolic rate,
- improve the ability of skeletal muscles to contract.

Coffee's pharmacological effects, in other words, amount to something of an Indianapolis 500 for your internal organs. Which might be acceptable if it adequately nourished you along the way. Or if you'd give your organs appropriate pit stops. But you don't. When you feel your first cup wearing off, you go for another. And coffee's insidious circle is off and rolling—given additional momentum by caffeine's tendencies to interfere with sleep and deplete the body of thiamine. Toss a jelly doughnut into the ring, and you've really got problems, because sugar, like caffeine, drives blood sugar too high, too fast. And the higher you go, the harder you fall.

But you may run into problems even before you have that second cup or jelly doughnut. Because you're sitting at your desk all day, you haven't got much of a chance to put coffee's physical effects to work. You have been "made ready" in many of the same ways, in fact, that our prehistoric ancestors were made ready by the likes of an angry beast. Adrenaline has been released. Your senses have been sharpened. But for what? Caffeine prepares us for action that in today's world usually never comes.

Unless, of course, we go around slamming file cabinets. "High doses of caffeine . . . can produce . . . symptoms that are indistinguishable from those of anxiety neurosis," writes John F. Greden, M.D., in the *American Journal of Psychiatry* (October, 1974). Nervousness, irritability, rapid heart rate and muscle twitchings can result from keeping too many coffee highs on hold.

But that's only part of it. "The post-stimulation letdown which can occur with caffeine results in fatigue and lethargy, and the constant stimulation caused by chronic caffeine usage could be disastrous," said Sanford Bolton, Ph.D., associate professor of pharmacy at St. John's University in Queens, New York (*Journal of*

Applied Nutrition, Spring, 1981). In short, zapping your body with caffeine wears it down. Depression may even follow in some cases. You probably already know that too much caffeine can also deprive you of a good night's sleep—running you down even further. But did you know you can have difficulty sleeping after you *stop* drinking coffee regularly? Caffeine also affects the calcium in muscles—which can affect muscle stamina. (See the chapter Vitamins and Minerals that Combat Fatigue.) And caffeine enhances the absorption and metabolism of drugs—some of which may cause fatigue in themselves.

So does that mean you should stop drinking coffee altogether? It's worth a try. Or at least keep it down to one morning cup. If that's too much for you, see the section How Some of Us Wake Up in the chapter Wake Up Feeling Fresher for other ways to get yourself going in the morning.

Cigarettes Fog Your Brain

Like the caffeine in coffee, the nicotine in cigarettes stimulates the central nervous system. Adrenaline is summoned and the heart beats faster. But. . . .

The carbon monoxide in cigarette smoke reduces the ability of the blood to carry oxygen, with the result being a *decreased* oxygen supply to serve the heart's *increased* oxygen demand. It's a very fatiguing situation for the body, and one that's tiring for the brain, as well.

But you say you need a smoke to help you think? Recently a clinical psychologist at the University of Edinburgh in Scotland gave a memory test to 37 smokers and 37 nonsmokers selected at random. They were to remember the names of 12 people shown to them in photographs. The smokers (good for an average of 20 cigarettes a day for at least 27 years) could recall an average of less than seven names, while the nonsmokers could remember an average of nearly nine (*British Medical Journal,* December 22-29, 1979).

People will tell you that smoking calms them, that it helps them work, that it does positive things for them—and that's why they smoke, Columbia University psychologist Stanley Schachter, Ph.D., has observed. What they fail to reveal, however, is that they climb the walls when they can't. "The heavy smoker gets nothing out of smoking. He smokes only to prevent withdrawal" (*Annals of Internal Medicine,* January, 1978). Nicotine is a powerfully addictive drug.

And like caffeine, nicotine interferes with sleep. In a two-part study at Penn State's Sleep Research and Treatment Center in

Hershey, Pennsylvania, it was discovered that while it took an average of 30 minutes for a group of 50 nonsmokers to fall asleep, a group of 50 smokers took roughly 44 minutes. What's more, when 8 smokers (who had been smoking between 30 and 60 cigarettes a day for at least two years) were made to quit cold turkey, the time it took them to fall asleep decreased by 65 percent in the first three nights—and continued to drop at a slightly slower rate during the next six (*Science,* February 1, 1980).

Alcohol: an Energy Hoax

Which brings us to the subject of nightcaps. Putting a tight one on every evening is *not* the way to wake up raring to go. Alcohol has been shown in laboratory experiments to shorten the amount of time imbibers spend in REM (rapid eye movement) sleep, the all-important stage during which we dream. And sleeping pills have been shown to do the same thing.

Alcohol as a "lift" during the day poses a different set of problems. Pharmacologically speaking, alcohol is not a stimulant, but rather a central nervous system depressant. It might *feel* stimulating, but that's only because it's depressing your inhibitions and encouraging you to expend more energy than perhaps you should.

Some Natural Alternatives. . .

If you rely on coffee, alcohol and cigarettes for regular pick-me-ups, we suggest that you cut down (or better yet, give up) one at a time to gradually lessen their roller coaster impact. And for a lift that lasts, turn to healthier eating habits, an exercise program, a renewed hobby—even a new outlook on life. Let's be a little more specific.

FOOD. In a study done several years ago, it was found that out of a group of 78 people complaining of fatigue and fluid retention—all of whom normally skipped breakfast—58 were helped markedly when they ate a high-protein meal in the morning. They were advised to include as part of their breakfast one or more of the following: four to five egg whites, fish, meat or cheese (mozzarella, cottage or provolone), or flavored gelatins with the addition of at least two tablespoons of brewer's yeast. They were also advised to reduce their intake of refined carbohydrates—meaning sugar, white bread and processed cereal (*Medical Tribune,* April, 1976).

Why?

Because proteins do not cause the rapid rises in blood sugar that sugars and refined carbohydrates do. And it is these rapid rises that lead to rapid crashes as the pancreas panics in response to sugar overloads, pouring out more sugar-taming insulin than it should.

High-protein snacks *during* the day might also be a good idea. Try them in place of sweet nothings from the vending machine. (For more details, see the chapter Eating for Daylong Energy.)

EXERCISE. Exercise stimulates many of the same adrenal responses as caffeine and nicotine—but at a rate you can live with. It also rejuvenates your blood's supplies of oxygen and releases mood-elevating chemicals in the brain. So try a few jumping jacks the next time the eyelids are at half-mast. And in the event you aren't already, get yourself on a regular fitness program. Considering exercise was our way of life for millions of years, it should come as no surprise that depression and fatigue are often the result of not getting enough. (See the chapter Energize with Exercise for more on the stimulating powers of exertion.)

FUN. Easier said than done. But think about it, anyway. If your career is wearing you down, *despite* an otherwise healthy life-style, your future in that career is not a good one.

Your fatigue could be due to either frustration, confusion or disinterest. And the best cure for that kind of tiredness is clear sight of a desired goal. Just ask any marathoner how it feels to be within eyesight of the finish. (See also Part 3, Make Time for Fun.)

PART III

Make Time for Fun

Are You a Workaholic?

CHAPTER7

Do you find it impossible to pass a messy room without rushing in to clean it up? Do you feel guilty if you don't arrive early at work? Do you always volunteer for extra jobs? Are you making more and more lists so that you won't forget ordinary things? Are you thinking of taking on a second job? Has anyone ever called you a workaholic?

Until now, we've discussed ways to help you get going. But maybe you have the opposite problem. You see, it's equally important to be able to stop what you're doing in order to periodically recoup your energies. If not, you can end up *awfully* pooped.

"Workaholics are people who just don't know when to stop working," said John M. Rhoads, M.D., professor of psychiatry at Duke University Medical Center. "Some people seem to lack an inner monitoring device for regulating the work-rest-recreation balance. Plagued by a compulsive need to work, they deny the existence of fatigue and push themselves beyond reason. Workaholics are the sort of people who lengthen their workday to compensate for their lessened ability to produce, which only accentuates the problem. They not only become more tired but they also eliminate exercise or recreation time, further diminishing their recuperative capacity.

"The 'work ethic' is probably the culprit here," continued Dr. Rhoads. "It's striking that in my field there are few articles dealing specifically with problems of overwork, but by contrast a large number dealing with the inability or unwillingness to work.

Apparently we are all so agreed on the inherent sinfulness of laziness that we overlook even the obsessive causes of overwork."

All Kinds of Workaholics

That people in high-pressure, high-powered executive jobs are often workaholics is well known. Not so well known is that many ordinary people, from schoolkids to housewives and elderly people, can be workaholics, too.

"Everyone is susceptible," said Dr. Rhoads, who has conducted two ground-breaking studies on workaholism. "Compulsive absorption in work may be brought on by many kinds of pressure. It may be emotional problems or it may be money problems or a tough deadline. Suddenly you have to really put your nose to the grindstone, work longer hours, work on weekends, neglect your family, friends and other activities. We all have to do that sometimes. It becomes a problem only when it becomes habitual."

Once workaholic behavior becomes habitual, the early symptoms that we mentioned become more severe. Workaholics typically suffer from a variety of psychosomatic illnesses such as anxiety reactions and heart, circulation and stomach ailments. These are not imaginary maladies, like the diseases of the hypochondriac, but very real medical problems. In many cases, they drive the workaholic to drug dependency on tranquilizers or obsessive reliance on cigarettes or alcohol.

In Dr. Rhoads's first study of workaholics, he presented a typical case: a 39-year-old housewife and mill worker who finally sought psychiatric help when she came down with not only chronic fatigue, but excruciating headaches, crying spells, weight loss and constipation. When the results of physical and laboratory tests showed that she was not suffering from any disease, Dr. Rhoads questioned her about her work habits.

He discovered that she was known to all her friends as a fanatical housekeeper. Rather than ask her daughter to iron her own clothes and clean up her own room, the housewife felt compelled to do it herself. "I know she's taking advantage of me," Dr. Rhoads's patient told him, "but I can't stand to pass the room and see the mess." The woman was also unable to keep a maid—even with her two jobs—because she couldn't tolerate tasks that weren't done perfectly. Her family insisted that the house was clean enough, but that couldn't dissuade the woman from her compulsive cleaning (*Journal of the American Medical Association,* June 13, 1977).

Ironically, work addiction sometimes breeds the same inefficiency that the workaholic loathes. Reluctance to delegate work and a compulsive need for things to be perfect—two prime workaholic characteristics—can undermine the effectiveness of even the busiest of work addicts. One M.D., in fact, asserted that the notion of the workaholic being efficient is a myth. "It takes him 12 hours to do what others can do in only 8."

Students can easily become workaholics, too, said another doctor. "Students . . . frequently suffer similar difficulties as they attempt to 'do their best' without having a realistic definition of just what their 'best' should be," wrote James C. Sams, M.D., of Scottsville, Virginia, in response to Dr. Rhoads's study. The misconception of the schoolchild "and especially the college student as one who has limitless energy and abundant rest and recreation may cause the unwary physician to fail to consider the possibility of overwork as a cause for vague symptoms in this age group and may result in a spurious [false] diagnosis of mononucleosis" (*Journal of the American Medical Association*, October 10, 1977).

One might naturally assume that as people approach their later years, they would look forward to taking it easy. That's not necessarily the case, though. Dr. Rhoads reports that some elderly people who cannot accept the physical limitations of poor health or aging may turn to obsessive work to prove their continuing worth in the form our society most readily recognizes. "One often finds such persons in their sixties attempting to maintain their schedule of 40 years ago," he says. "That would be fine if they could handle it. But that's precisely the problem with the workaholic, young or old: he doesn't know how to handle a busy schedule. He goes too hard for too long, and that takes its toll."

Let Up on the Gas

Workaholism is well illustrated in remarks by some of the workaholics in Dr. Rhoads's study. One man, a 55-year-old attorney who never worked less than 65 hours a week and had not taken a vacation for five years, felt guilty if he felt tired. If he left work early or didn't go in early, he also suffered from a guilty conscience. "I feel sinful if I'm not working," he told Dr. Rhoads. When advised to relax and take a holiday, another workaholic said, "Fun is something you have to learn to do by working hard at it."

"Workaholics are commonly attempting to solve life's problems by excessive, distracting work," explained Dr. Rhoads.

"Overwork may represent an effort to maintain a clear conscience by saying to the world, 'See, I am blameless. I have done all that I could, even working to the edge of total exhaustion.' "

When workaholism is habitual and shows the more severe symptoms, its victim needs to be reoriented to be made aware of his physical and emotional requirements and attend to them. That involves helping him understand the origins of his work compulsion and counseling him with respect to future work patterns.

In mild cases of workaholism, a vacation and counseling may be all that is required. Dr. Rhoads has sometimes even taken advantage of the compulsive nature of workaholics to set up a rigid schedule of rest and recreation.

Other doctors take a similar approach. "People come here and I tell them they must stop working right *now*," said Jose A. Yaryura-Tobias, M.D., medical director of Bio-Behavioral Psychiatry in Great Neck, New York. Dr. Yaryura-Tobias describes our need for regular, frequent "pit stops" in terms of what he calls brain fatigue.

"The brain tires like a muscle," explained Dr. Yaryura-Tobias. "When a muscle is fatigued, it gives you a signal, pain or cramps, which is due to the lack of oxygen in the muscle. You have to rest to recover. The brain will also give you signals when it is overtired—inability to concentrate, inability to put thoughts together, a sense of irritability to minor things. You feel jumpy, nervous. You may have difficulty in falling asleep or staying asleep. You go from lows to highs. The brain cannot control itself any longer. The brain works by excitation and inhibition. When there is fatigue, those things begin to be altered, and they do not coordinate. The incoordination of the brain will bring incoordination of the thought process, in the mood, in intellectual capacity—in all the functions that you have."

For most of us brain fatigue is part of our normal daily cycle. But then we eat a good dinner, read a book, do some exercises. We have switched from doing one thing to another that is unrelated, and that rests the brain so we are ready for the next day's work load. But for many others, brain fatigue becomes a chronic condition. Fatigue builds upon fatigue with no recovery period in between. You can't catch up with just a night's sleep anymore. You find yourself unable to concentrate or put thoughts together. You have pushed yourself to an extreme and you can't return any longer.

"Unfortunately, because brain fatigue is not a visual thing no one believes it exists, not even the patients who are describing the symptoms," said Dr. Yaryura-Tobias. "They keep on trying to work, and to do that they take stimulants—coffee and amphet-amines. They go out at night and have cocktails. A lot of them are on tranquilizers and sleeping pills. They do all that because without it they could not function.

"By the time they come in for a consultation they may have a drug problem to go along with the brain fatigue. That is when I feel the nutritional approach is best, along with resting the brain. We give supplements, especially the B complex vitamins, and a program of exercises along with a good diet. Physical exercise is very important, too. It is one of the most perfect things to reduce anxiety and tension." (See Part 2, Supernutrition for Work and Play, for more information on diet and fatigue.)

"When I recommend physical exercise and nutrition, it's not for one week—it's forever," pointed out Dr. Yaryura-Tobias. "It's a lifestyle that one has to adopt permanently to remain in good mental health."

Dr. Sams best sums it up this way: "I have found it useful to compare overwork and decreased efficiency to a finely tuned automobile spinning its wheels in the snow: the need is not to burn more fuel, race the engine faster, and dig in deeper, but to let up on the gas so that normal progress can resume."

Workaholic or Good Worker?

But letting up on the gas is not the same as letting the car idle. A hard worker, who enjoys his job and is dedicated to it, is not the same as a workaholic. "Long hours of work are not what make one ill," said Dr. Rhoads. "If the work is enjoyed and provides a reasonable amount of freedom, there is no good reason for an individual to become ill. But the crucial factor is certain personality features that enable the individual to cope."

To determine what precisely distinguishes the healthy, hard worker from the workaholic, Dr. Rhoads conducted a follow-up study with 15 "effective, successful, physically and mentally healthy" workers who thrive on extremely long schedules (at least 60 hours a week). Those volunteers answered a questionnaire about lifestyle, attitude toward work and personal attributes. Dr. Rhoads compared the results with data from his study of workaholics.

"The most striking personality feature of the healthy, hard workers in contrast to the workaholics is that they know when to stop. They could spot fatigue and respond to it promptly. Most respond by quitting work early or taking time off. They schedule and enjoy vacations, spend time with their families, keep up with their friendships, and exercise regularly. In short, they have other outlets for their drive besides work."

Learning to Love Leisure

By contrast, one psychiatrist has described workaholics as "leisure neurotics." And another leisure consultant explained what that means. "It may sound silly, but some people don't like time away from the work routine," said Richard Kraus, Ed.D., chairman of Temple University's department of recreation and leisure, in Philadelphia. "They can't adjust to having free time and using it properly. On weekends, they virtually break down. In very extreme cases, they may take trips, but after a day or two—even a day or two in Europe—they fly back. Leisure implies a kind of personal freedom and they can't deal with that. They can't leave the security of their job's routine. Work for them is a structured, organized, socially approved activity with a clear outcome."

The prospect of unfilled, unscheduled time can be scary. "A good instance of how scary the freedom of leisure time can be is that in a work-obsessed society such as ours we tend to organize our leisure," Dr. Kraus said. "We schedule ourselves for leisure time: we take classes and learn 'leisure skills'; we compete and we gain status through our play. Obligation is an important factor—we have commitments to the community band, the bowling league and the Girl Scout troop.

"The original meaning of leisure, on the other hand, implied that it was time for freedom, contemplation, choice, and was not necessarily structured, purposeful or even constructive. Leisure is more ambiguous than work, with a wider range of choices and outcomes. It's very hard for someone who has the kind of rigid personality one observes in workaholics to accept the freedom."

For more on how to truly enjoy your leisure time, read the next two chapters: 15 Reasons Why You Should Take a Vacation, and Never Be Bored Again.

15 Reasons Why You Should Take a Vacation

CHAPTER 8

We've all heard that vacations are important. But what exactly can they do for our energy levels? Is it worth the time, trouble and expense to interrupt our lives and take off somewhere? Or will we come back more tired than when we left? The answers are: (1) vacations can do a *lot* for our energy levels, (2) they're *definitely* worth the time and expense and (3) we won't really come back more tired.

Let's back up. Sure, you'll feel a little tuckered out after a trip. But it's a rejuvenating kind of energy expenditure, unlike the life-weariness that you started out with. So in the long run, yes, it's definitely worth it. Your vacation is going to give you a boost in many different ways. At least 15, by our count.

1. Relaxation

"Just the act of getting away from your daily frustrations will relax you," said Richard I. Curtis, author of *Taking Off* (Harmony, 1981). "Even if you come up against some new problems on your trip, you can treat these like a game. They're temporary. The important thing is, you are getting out of your day-to-day rut," Curtis told us.

Edward Heath, Ph.D., professor in the department of recreation and parks of Texas A & M University, agreed:

"When you take a vacation, you escape the humdrum of daily life. You leave your troubles behind you. Even if all you do is sit on the edge of the river and watch a rock move, it's a valuable change of pace. You're going to recharge your batteries. You'll return refreshed and renewed."

2. Stimulation of New Sights

Richard Curtis told us, "almost any travel is good. Staying at home for too long tends to crimp our awareness. We need the exposure to new sights and experiences. Think of the first time you saw mountains, or the sea, or the desert, or the Grand Canyon—I don't mean pictures. I mean actually being there, in a place that is totally different from anything you're used to."

New sights of things around us can give us new insights, too, according to Dr. Heath. "You can get a broader view, a new perspective on your own world, if you visit a different place. For example, if you live at the mouth of the Mississippi or the Hudson, or some other great river, you may understand your own region better after visiting the headwaters of the river. You may learn something about yourself, too—namely, that you might like to move to that new area. Lots of people take advantage of their vacations to look over other regions they might like to move to someday."

3. Meeting New People

"We're very social animals," Dr. Heath said. "A vacation gives us the opportunity to form new friendships—or just to satisfy our curiosity about how other people live. This gives us a broader perspective on our own lives."

Richard Curtis agreed: "The more people you know, the more eyes you can borrow to look on the world. And the further those eyes are from your own world, the better."

4. Fellowship and Camaraderie

"Sharing an adventure with other people allows us to share their enthusiasm, too. That's good. It's positive reinforcement for our own enthusiasm about life," Dr. Heath said. "But it doesn't necessarily have to be easy going. Shared hardships also form bonds of love and friendship and give us something to look back on with pride and pleasure.

"Twenty years from now, you'll remember and talk about the canoe trip where the weather suddenly changed and you spent two days huddled over a campfire, shivering.

"There's also a benefit in associating with like-minded people in some competitive event," said Dr. Heath. "People travel thousands of miles to cheer their team in the Super Bowl or the playoffs. Marathon runners travel halfway across the world to run in a race and be surrounded by thousands of other runners."

5. Education

"You may need or want to learn new skills on your vacation," Dr. Heath said. "You may decide to learn a new language before traveling to a foreign country. Or you may learn as you go along in order to communicate with people there. You may decide to learn snorkeling, or tennis, or golf, or skiing, or mountain climbing, or hang gliding or any new skill."

6. Adventure

"Travel returns a sense of adventure to your life," said Curtis. "Pulling yourself off your native turf is going to make demands on your resourcefulness—to find suitable lodging and food. But you're also allowed to experiment with your personality and lifestyle without having to live with the consequences. If you're usually too shy to say hello and smile at strangers, you may allow yourself the adventure of doing just that on your vacation in a new place. It may then become a habit you can bring home with you."

The element of risk is also a part of many vacation adventures, according to Dr. Heath. "Most travel involves accepting and meeting challenges. You test yourself against a new environment. You can improve your self-esteem by taking on challenges that everyday life doesn't offer. Of course, sometimes everyday life may involve greater risk. Waterskiing, mountain climbing, skydiving—all seem quite scary. But though they may be more thrilling, they actually are safer than driving on the freeway."

7. Surprise

"It is the unexpected in life that we learn from," said Curtis. "We gain the most when we put ourselves on the line and remain open to new experiences. On a trip you have to adapt very quickly. You bring much of that enhanced adaptability home with you." Not to mention the stories of all your surprises, which you'll remember for many years.

8. Beauty

"When you're standing in the middle of a beautiful environment, and you open your eyes to it, you start to feel in tune with it. You can actually begin to feel beautiful yourself. You share some of the beauty and power," Dr. Heath told us. "You may have such a peak experience in a natural setting, like the Grand Canyon—or your awe might be inspired by the beauty of some man-made edifice such as the Vatican, or a bridge, or a whole city.

"These experiences we never forget are very important to our enjoyment of life."

9. Anticipation

Have we got you itchin' to hit the road for action and adventure and new people, places and things? Are you so excited you can't wait to plan your vacation? Good, because that's part of the benefit of a vacation. "Your vacation," according to Dr. Heath, "is more than the actual time spent away from home. The planning and preparation are also good for you. Many vacations are actually yearlong projects. A person may prepare for a fishing trip, for example, by tying flies. The anticipation is pleasurable. The trip is, too, because you reap the rewards of extensive preparation."

10. Memories

"Your life is enriched before, during and after a vacation," Dr. Heath said. "You'll always have the joy of reflecting on pleasant memories."

11. Freedom

"A vacation gives us the freedom to do what we want to do," added Dr. Heath.

"Our bodies have the remarkable ability to recognize a deficiency and try to compensate for it," noted Curtis. "The mind, too, seems to have a myriad of ways to deal with psychological problems without necessarily consulting the brain's owner. Our desire for change occurs regularly. Even if you are generally satisfied with your life and work, you may still feel the need for something more. You may feel closed in. Take a vacation and you will realize your own freedom. You'll see that the mundane world can be transcended at will. It can be left behind. You're not a prisoner if you choose not to be."

12. Self-Discovery

"A vacation can be a great opportunity for sorting out life's experiences," Dr. Heath told us. "You can shut off the sensory overload that may be your everyday life and get away to a deserted beach or a mountain stream.

"You can let your soul talk to itself. The dialogue you carry on with yourself is very important. You need it to develop your creativity and your inner peace and harmony."

13. Appreciation of Things Taken for Granted

"You'll be surprised at the things for which you become homesick," Curtis said. "You'll crave the simple pleasure of finding someone who speaks your language. I have felt almost sick for the sight of a lilac, for a maple tree, for ice cream sodas, for a long, hot shower and even—I hate to admit it—for American fast food. I once ran alongside an American's car for three blocks in Yugoslavia—just to hear an old Simon and Garfunkel song on his tape player.

"When you get home, you will get more from life. You'll see the miracles where you live."

14. Time Stands Still

"If you're really enjoying yourself," Dr. Heath said, "time does not progress in equal units. You stop thinking about everything else but what you're doing then and there.

"You get lost in the activity of the moment. You may be catching fish, or trying to keep dry while canoeing through the rapids, or looking for pretty shells along the beach.

"Time is standing still for you and that's good. There's evidence that happy people are those who can give full attention to what's going on at that moment."

15. Happiness

We saved the most important reason for last. "The major goal of a vacation is happiness," said Dr. Heath. "Your leisure time should make you happier. A vacation is not a necessary evil you endure to enable you to work harder when you get back. Your leisure makes up a large segment of your life, and it can and should be a valuable force for good. You should like your life a little better after a vacation."

Never Be Bored Again

CHAPTER 9

If you're tired, that doesn't necessarily mean you have no energy. You might simply be bored.

Let's put it another way: ever notice how children are always eager to try new things or continue to play long after Mom, Dad or the babysitter has run out of steam? Part of the reason for the seemingly endless energy of children is that they haven't been weighted down with years of accumulated tension, responsibility and commitments. For adults, on the other hand, it's easy to slip into tedium. Day in and day out, we get up, shower, eat, drink, go to work, meet deadlines, come home, clean, pay bills, cook and so on. With the loss of spontaneity, our routine begins to weigh us down. The fact is, boredom is yet another major cause of fatigue.

But it's never too late to snap out of that edgy, irritable feeling and rekindle the childlike curiosity and enthusiasm for life within each of us. Now, that doesn't mean totally abandoning our jobs and other commitments to loll around in a grass hut somewhere. But taking some time to develop our interests, our sense of humor, and our creativity goes a long way toward cultivating what the French call *joie de vivre*—joy of living. You might say *joie de vivre* is the opposite of boredom.

How can we avoid boredom? By recognizing it, and then *doing* something about it.

"We have to recognize first of all that boredom is a nearly universal experience," said Robert Plutchik, Ph.D., a professor of psychiatry and psychology at the Albert Einstein College of Medicine in New York City and author of *Emotion: A Psycho-evolutionary Synthesis* (Harper & Row, 1980). "Everybody has **79** experienced boredom because it represents an expression of what I call a 'basic emotion.' "

According to Dr. Plutchik, to get rid of boredom you should seek an interest in something relevant to your own life. "For instance, many people start out indifferent to nutritional issues," he said. "Then, when they are older or have an illness, they develop an intense interest—because they see the relevance of nutrition to their own life."

Along the same lines, New York City psychoanalyst Theodore Rubin, M.D., believes that, when it comes to developing interests, we have to get our feet wet before we can enjoy the swim. "In an attempt to mitigate boredom I find it of great value to remember that *involvement precedes interest*," he said. "We must risk at least a minimum degree of involvement in any activity or enterprise before interest can be generated. Waiting for an interest to strike us before we take steps to become involved may well keep us in a state of relative boredom for a lifetime."

The Joy of Learning

What activity should you pick? "Learning, with its implication of newness, open-endedness, self-achievement and pride—with its promise of mastery—is the greatest antidote to boredom," said Willard Gaylin, M.D., a psychiatrist from New York City.

Dr. Rubin seconds the motion. "It is just about never too late to go back to books, to take courses, to attend lectures, to develop a latent interest. Boredom simply cannot exist when we are actively engaged in the process of continuing growth through recognition and development of real resources in ourselves."

Using Both Sides of Your Brain

Learning doesn't have to be drudgery. It can be fun—an easy, joyful process of opening your life to new interests and expertise—*if* you get your entire brain in on the act.

And the first step is to use *both sides* of your brain.

Over the last 20 years, scientific research has shown that the brain has two sides, or hemispheres, and that they function very differently.

"Most classroom teaching only makes use of the left hemisphere," said Owen Caskey, Ed.D., professor of education and psychology at Texas Tech University. The left hemisphere, he explained, works with facts—logical, point-by-point thinking. But the right hemisphere works with feeling—fantasy, imagination, mental imagery and intuition.

"And when both hemispheres of the brain are involved in

learning," said Don Schuster, Ph.D., professor of psychology at Iowa State University, "learning is easier, faster and much more fun."

Dr. Schuster "trains" people by having them use success goal imagery to overcome a major block to learning—the fear of difficulty and failure. "A person who expects that learning can be easy will learn easily, and enjoy it in the process," he said. "I instruct people to picture themselves mastering material and having fun doing it. For instance, a student will picture himself sitting at a desk with a book and a smile on his face."

Dr. Schuster believes most people, unfortunately, develop the idea when they're very young that they can't learn easily—and so they go through life accepting other people's evaluation of their learning ability. As we approach our later years, that misconception is often reinforced. "In older people, there is the fear that the mind can't remember as well as it used to," said Carl Schleicher, Ph.D., director of Mankind Research Unlimited, a Silver Spring, Maryland, organization that offers classes to develop learning skills. "But there is no need for stress and mental pain while learning. People have been brainwashed to accept limitations. The mind is unlimited in its capacity to learn—the only limitations are those that have been imposed on us or that we impose on ourselves."

Tips for Learning Faster and Easier

To free the mind of fear and anxiety, Dr. Schleicher—and every other education expert we talked to—emphasized the necessity of a relaxation technique. Dr. Caskey told us, "A relaxation skill is the most crucial element to improve learning ability. Anxiety interferes with learning. *Any* kind of anxiety, not just that type associated with the learning process itself. If you can rid an individual of anxiety, he is more likely to learn." (See the chapter Lighten Up with Relaxation for simple relaxation methods that work.)

While relaxation helps you prepare to learn something new, listening to music *while* studying is also very calming, said Dr. Schuster.

"Reviewing material while listening to baroque music—music that has approximately one beat per second, such as quite a bit of music by Bach, Handel and Vivaldi—helps keep you in a relaxed state of mind."

Dr. Caskey thinks that any soothing music will do. "Unhurried, stately music makes a wonderful background for studying," he said. "We use both classical music and the type of music you hear on 'easy listening' FM radio."

Jane Bancroft, Ph.D., professor of French at the University of Toronto, was one of the first people to conduct studies on music and learning.

"I first became interested in methods to enhance memory and concentration when I realized that year by year my students were becoming poorer in their ability to learn French," she told us. "After thorough research, I attribute this trend to two main factors: the influence of television, which trains attention to be passive and dull, and the increase of junk food and additives in the diet.

"Right diet is one of the basics of good memory," she continued. "If you don't eat properly, you don't nourish the brain. A colleague of mine came to the U.S. and stayed in a typical chain hotel, eating most of her meals in the restaurant there. After a few days, she remarked that her mind wasn't as sharp as usual. I think it was because the food served in such restaurants is often processed and loaded with additives."

But, says Dr. Bancroft, the brain isn't nourished only by food. "If a person sits in a cramped position in a windowless room with no fresh air, he's not going to be able to concentrate or memorize well because his brain isn't getting enough oxygen. Deep, rhythmic breathing during a study session is very helpful to maintain an alert, relaxed state of mind."

And if you use one or many of these techniques—relaxation, restful music, good diet and deep breathing—to learn, you may find that not only your learning ability, but also your "livability" improves, too.

"People are better able to accept and learn from the challenges of life when they use more of their brain," said Barbara McNeill, a wellness educator from Mill Valley, California. "Life is learning," she told us. "You can't separate the two. A person who is healthy and happy is someone who knows how to learn from life."

Have a Good Laugh

A few good laughs are a rousing anthem to the soul.

Several doctors and psychologists we spoke to made some encouraging comments about the relationship among a sense of humor, our health and our general enthusiasm for life.

"I find it draining to be around serious-minded people all the time," said David E. Bresler, Ph.D., of the University of California at Los Angeles Medical Center. "Uplifting people uplift others."

We all know people who were brought up without positive reinforcement of their funny bone, while others seem to find humor even in the most serious of situations.

"Eliminate the negative people," suggested other health professionals we spoke with. "Surround yourself with the positive ones—people who fill you with joy and laughter, rather than gloom and doom."

Harry A. Olson, Ph.D., calls that "modeling," and it's one of the fastest ways to develop a positive sense of humor. "Humor cannot be taught systematically," said Dr. Olson, a psychologist from Reisterstown, Maryland, "but must be observed and personally experienced to be mastered."

When's the last time you had a good hearty belly laugh? You know—the kind where your whole body gets involved. You find yourself thrown against the back of your chair one minute, and then doubled over the next. Great loud noises burst from your upturned and opened mouth. Tears flow from the corners of your eyes, and you grasp the sides of your body in mock agony. At the same time, tense muscles go limp—so much so that at the height of your enjoyment you may not even have the strength to make a fist.

Come to think of it, good, hearty laughter is a lot like exercise—it aids the circulation, massages the abdominal muscles, stimulates digestion, lowers blood pressure, and "begets optimism and self-confidence and relegates fear and pessimism to the background." So wrote E. Forrest Boyd, M.D., back in the 40s (*Southwestern Medicine,* July, 1942). As such, laughter can rejuvenate you much the same as can a few minutes of stretching or a brisk walk.

While there are a lot of situations that may make you laugh, not all of them have uplifting qualities. "Humor as a therapeutic tool must build instead of knock, and therefore excludes sarcasm and cynicism, which pump up the self at the expense of others," said Dr. Olson.

The fact is, *why* you laugh is just as important as *how* you laugh.

"There are three levels of humor," explained Dr. Olson. "Sarcasm is one, but that's destructive. The second, a good pun that gives you a twist of expectancy, has positive qualities. And so does the third level, cosmic humor, which is an appreciation of the paradoxes and absurdities of life.

"The person who has this level of humor is more likely to be flexible and able to take in stride what life dishes out," said Dr. Olson. "I like level three the best for my patients."

So have a good laugh or two today. And while you're at it, make it a point to be good to yourself. That means doing something you especially enjoy and never have time for. Don't keep putting off fun until you have more time, finish this or that project, feel better, or whatever other excuse you can come up with.

How to Be Alone without Being Lonely

"Loneliness is often a synonym for boredom," said social psychology researcher Carin Rubenstein, Ph.D. "People who spend their time creatively when alone are learning to deal with solitude. They forget about their loneliness and begin feeling more calm, relaxed, creative and happy."

The art of being alone seems to have been ignored by some and abused by others in American society. Conflicts over how best to spend one's time can erupt as early as childhood.

"If a child sits staring at a dandelion for two minutes, some adult will come along and holler, 'What in blazes are you trying to do? Can't you find something to do with yourself?'" said Alexander Reid Martin, M.D., a former head of the American Psychiatric Association's Committee on Leisure. "What the adult fails to realize is that the child *is* doing something. But the sense of wonder, fascination and enterprise in his solitude is lost after the adult's intrusion.

"So many times we're at the mercy of those around us, who tell us what to do," said Dr. Martin. "So many times we are not left to our own inner resources. We're chased away from what we're doing and told to do something else."

Loneliness does not necessarily depend on the number of people around us or on life's varied circumstances, observed Dr. Rubenstein and co-worker Phillip Shaver, Ph.D., of New York University. Instead, it seems to be the result of how people interpret their situations. Loneliness is a combination of our personal expectations of life and our reactions to our environment. Eventually, the way we feel about being alone can alter. Apparently, the more time we spend alone, the more we get used to it.

"A person who is accustomed to living alone won't experience loneliness as much as others, since that person has learned how to cope with solitude," said Dr. Rubenstein. "Older people in their mid-sixties and seventies are much better adjusted to being alone than younger people. Their need for intimate attachments is less. And they are more likely to spend their time creatively when alone."

Making the Most of Time Spent Alone

Through their research, Drs. Rubenstein and Shaver discovered that when people feel lonely, they generally react in one of two ways. The "sad passivity" reaction means that the person is very passive when feeling lonely. Sleeping, eating and crying seem to be the three major activities in that camp.

The second reaction is "creative solitude," and many older adults fall into that bracket. When they feel lonely, they may read, listen to music, work on a hobby, study, write or play a musical instrument.

Dr. Martin stresses the phrase "inner resources," saying people should turn to "the god within" when they feel lonely. There they will find whatever they need to know in order to move forward with their lives.

"The word 'enthusiasm'," explained Dr. Martin, "comes from the root word 'entheos' which means 'the god within.' Enthusiasm for something cannot be superimposed on someone; it has to come from inside a person. I have seen some overly aggressive occupational workers in psychiatric hospitals poke, prod and push patients to try to get them enthused and involved in some new program. The patients just get stubborn and dig in their heels. Eventually, they may give in and take part only to please the worker. The therapist winds up happy, but the patient is bored to death."

Similar problems occur when someone is bereaved over the sudden death of a spouse. Dr. Martin believes friends and family should respect the person's right to mourn. After a while, the bereaved may be led back into the mainstream of life, but it must be done gradually and gently.

"It's difficult to rekindle enthusiasm in people who have experienced a serious loss," said Dr. Martin. "You must not push. You must let their enthusiasm light itself; you can't light it for them. That doesn't mean you should sit by and do nothing. Pay close attention to them. Be alert and listen to what they say. Their enthusiasm will not lie fallow long. See what it is that kindles their flame and sets them going.

"All of us were born with inner resources," he told us. "In order to be able to use our faculties, abilities and inventiveness in some constructive, creative way, we must rely on them," concluded Dr. Martin. "People will never feel lonely if they will turn to their god within."

Get to Know Yourself Better

"If you're suddenly left alone, you should see it as an opportunity to discover yourself," said David A. Chiriboga, Ph.D., associate professor of psychology at the University of California at San Francisco. "Take it as a challenge. Find out what you want to be, where you want to go and what gives you pleasure. Anyone is an interesting person if he lets himself be. All people have to do is to look inside themselves."

"Talking out loud to oneself privately is healthy and actually may be a better way of tackling problems than suffering in silence," said Murray Halfond, Ph.D., a professor of speech at Temple University in Philadelphia. "Saying things out loud when we're alone is a catharsis—a tension release. After all, we vocalize when we are under great stress. If we bang our thumb with a hammer, we may swear or say ouch. We do something to get the experience off our chest."

Dreams, meditation and diaries also can be effective forms of self-communication, said Dr. Halfond. "Diaries are good methods of self-communication if you write more than 'I swept the floor and made the beds today.' A diary should not dwell on a subject continuously but should record our thoughts and our interactions with others."

In one exercise, Dr. Halfond instructs his students to write a dialogue depicting themselves communicating with someone out of their past. "They don't have to read it or show it to anyone. The scripts can show the students' insights about themselves. People can also use a tape recorder to sound out their problems. Or they can record their daytime fantasies. We daydream or fantasize, but we never make any use of those thoughts. Our subconscious could be more important to us than our conscious self. We should tune into it."

"I Love Being Alone"

People who have learned to be content both with themselves and with others just can't lose. Ruth Mills of Santa Monica, California, is one of those people. At 91 years of age, Mrs. Mills hosts the radio show *The Art of Being Your Age* every Monday afternoon on station KCRW–FM. She says she interviews a lot of interesting people and really enjoys her job. She also indulges in a few other outside activities.

"I take one or two classes a semester at Santa Monica College. I just finished one on the Middle East. I enjoy playing bridge, and I have very interesting friends who enjoy talking about different things."

Since she lives with a daughter who is frequently away, Mrs. Mills has quite a bit of time to herself.

"I love being alone. It doesn't bother me in the least. I do a lot of sewing. I make some of my own clothes. I love to read biographies, and I keep up on the political events of the day. I do the housework and go for walks. And I know if I want to do something else I can. If people want to sit in a chair and rock, by golly, it's their privilege. But I would deteriorate if I did it.

"Oh, I have times when I could start feeling sorry for myself. It goes on a bit, but then I say, 'Now listen, that's enough of *that!*' " The command is issued in a voice suddenly reflecting all of the patience and compassion of a Marine drill sergeant. She stops speaking for a moment, then adds almost wistfully, "I just push those thoughts right out of my head and think, 'Isn't it wonderful that the sun is shining?' "

Of course, we realize that beating boredom may not always be as easy as simply telling yourself to "snap out of it." That's where developing the acquaintance of positive, uplifting people can help. And once you've gotten involved in one or more interests— learning to speak a foreign language, to play a musical instrument, to draw, or whatever—there'll hardly be room for loneliness or boredom in your life. Because in the course of building regular interludes of fun in your life, chances are you will find yourself approaching every day with high energy and enthusiasm.

•

Index